Legal & Disclaimer

The information contained in this book is not designed to replace or take the place of any form of medication or professional medical advice. The information in this book has been provided for educational and entertainment purposes only.

The information contained in this book has been compiled from sources deemed reliable, and it is accurate to the best of the Author's knowledge. However, the Author cannot guarantee its accuracy and validity so cannot be held liable for any errors or omissions. Changes are periodically made to this book. You must consult your doctor or get professional medical advice before using any of the suggested remedies, techniques, or information in this book.

Upon using the information contained in this book, you agree to hold harmless the Author from and against any damages, costs and expenses, including any legal fees, potentially resulting from the application of any of the information provided by this guide. This disclaimer applies to any damages or injury caused by the use and application, whether directly or indirectly, of any advice or information presented, whether for breach of contract, tort, negligence, personal injury, criminal intent, or under any other cause of action.

You agree to accept all the risks of using the information presented inside this book. You need to consult a professional medical practitioner in order to ensure you are both able & healthy enough to participate in this program.

Contents

Introduction

I have to tell you about this Ketogenic Diet, or as you may heard it called, "The Keto Diet", it can help solve no end of problems and can help you lose weight in the process. It may be relatively new compared to some other diets, but this is no fad. Can you believe it first started over 90 years ago, as a cure for epilepsy in children? It did start to lose its impact after a few years as the introduction of new medicines were just being released onto the market. But would you believe it, mother nature was actually doing a better job of relieving epilepsy than the new medications? Maybe, that is why it started to become popular again around 1994. What made it become noticed again, was when a young Charlie Abraham made an astonishing recovery from epilepsy seizures, he was having on a daily basis, so happy were his family with these results, they decided to start "The Charlie Foundation". No matter what they had tried previously to the Keto Diet, nothing had worked. Charlie had been on the diet for 5 years, and it was then that his seizures stopped. In this book, I will explain how you can benefit from the Keto Diet, not just to lose weight but totally transform your life.

Advisory Note:

I know you are excited to get to the details, but let me just give you some advice, as with any diet, you should always seek the advice of a doctor or physician before starting, especially if you are taking any medication or suffering from any ailments.

It is especially crucial for anyone with Type 1 Diabetes to seek medical supervision before taking part in the diet.

Chapter 1 – Keto Diet Outline

The Keto Diet like many others consists of a low carb intake. It is these carbs which help the body produce energy, and the brain is fed chemicals which stimulate the pleasure centers. It is this that makes us feel happy by eating high carb foods. It should be mentioned, though, out of all the foods, it is nearly always carbs which cause the problems. They may give us a quick boost in energy, and stimulate the brain's pleasure centers, but there is one major downside to this, any carbs the body has not used to produce energy gets stored, and you guessed it, it gets stored as fat.

Now you may be thinking if carbs provide the energy, and we are about to consume fewer carbs, where will the body get energy from? Well, remember all the left-over carbs which are probably sitting on your belly? This will be the body's new energy source, or at least it will contribute towards it.

Chapter 2 – How the Keto Diet Works

The Keto diet principles are quite simple, we reduce the carbs and replace these by fats and proteins, this will after a while put the body into a state of Ketosis. It is in this state that the body burns ketones to produce energy rather than carbs. This simple process will lead us to weight loss and better health. I would like to mention, there are similar diets to this which are quite famous. Have you heard of the Atkins Diet? At least with the Keto Diet, you know it is based on scientific evidence that has been gathered over a period of nearly 100 years.

As discovered by Dr. Henry Rawle Geyelin, when a body is in a state of fasting, glucose levels contained in the blood drops, whilst at the same time, the levels of Ketones increases. When the body burns ketones for fuel rather than glucose, there is less stress on the brain, this is what reduces the onset of epileptic seizures.

Enough of the history lesson, let me explain how it works: When carbs are consumed in foods, they are converted into glucose, and it is this glucose which is the energy source to power the body and the brain in the bloodstream. Now the body is in a state of Ketosis, the liver will convert fats into fatty acids and ketones which can be used as a replacement for glucose to produce energy.

For the body to reach this state of ketosis, the majority of what is eaten should contain a high fat and protein content. As the number of carbs is restricted to around 50g per day, a lot of the vegetables that are grown above ground will have to be restricted, but your body will soon become super-efficient at burning fat for energy.

Studies have also shown, once the body is in a state of ketosis it can run 70% more efficiently as these ketones are actually preferred by the body over carbs.

Once on the diet, the first target is to deplete the bodies Glycogen stores, these are the way the body processes and stores glucose as energy, when you do high intensity activities like running, the muscles draw upon the glycogen for fuel, it is for this reason long distance runners do "carb loading" before big events.

In the liver, it is the glycogen that keeps the body functioning correctly all day, this includes the brain function, kidney cells and red blood cells.

Glycogen depletion is normally brought on by switching to a low carb diet like the Keto diet, it is in the first few days where you feel the side effects as mentioned, to fully deplete the glycogen stocks normally takes 2 -3 days on average. Each gram of glycogen is bound to 3-4 grams of water, so not only will you be depleting your glycogen stocks, there will be excess water being flushed from your system.

When first starting the Keto diet, counting calories is not what you should be concerned with, this is one of the reasons people start to lose interest and quit. The recipes supplied are structured to offer the best basis of how to achieve your goals.

Snacks

Not only is there recipes for breakfast, lunch and dinner, there are also plenty of snack recipes included that you can have to support your main meals, all these have been supplied to help you keep that full feeling so you have less intention of giving up, although the snack recipes are arranged for each week, it is possible to mix and match these for when you feel like them.

There are sumptuous smoothies, to one cup brownies, chips for a night on the sofa and many more. There are even popsicles and an easy to make ice cream that will stop you feeling deprived in any way.

As with the main meals, most have a limited carb count which should help you to reach a state of Ketosis in the quickest way with the minimum of effort, even these can be mixed and matched if so desired, the choice is yours.

Exercise

Strictly speaking there is no reason, why you need to exercise whilst on the Keto diet, to lose weight, the diet will do all the work. Although there are other benefits of exercise most of which are beneficial to your health:

Improved bone mineral density - studies show that resistance training improves bone mineral density in obese postmenopausal women.

Improved immunity - exercise may help you boost your immune system. Keep in mind that over exercising will have the opposite effect.

Improving diabetes by increasing insulin sensitivity - moderate aerobic exercise lowers blood sugar, the addition of one 10-second sprint after moderate intensity aerobic exercise can reduce hypoglycemia risk in physically active individuals who possess type 1 diabetes.

Brain health - exercise improves age-related cognitive decline and helps prevent neurodegenerative diseases.

Cardiovascular health - both vigorous and moderate physical activity help prevent coronary heart diseases.

Anti-ageing benefits - exercise may increase life expectancy by decreasing mortality risk factors like high blood pressure, type 2 diabetes, coronary heart disease, stroke and cancer.

You should not exercise just for the sake of burning calories to aid in weight loss, exercise should be done to promote muscle tone and help you feel good about yourself, so whatever activity you do, do it for pleasure.

If you contemplate any exercise, you should allow for plenty of rest between sessions, due to the lack of carbs, you may overdo it and be prone to dizzy spells until you have become accustomed to the diet properly.

Dining Out

Dining out especially at fast food joints could seem a bit daunting, but you have options that you may not realize you had. I will run through some of the more common places, and what is available for you.

McDonalds / Burger King

Both McDonald's and Burger King offer items that can be made low carb at a cheap price, you can ask for a breakfast sandwich at either restaurant and order without the bun the same goes for a grilled chicken breast or burger for a lunch or dinner. My personal favorite is the McDouble from McDonald's Value Menu, just forget the bun and the ketchup, very tasty and keto-friendly at only 4g carbs.

KFC

KFC is a great place to stop for a meal, each serving of their grilled chicken is either only 0 or 1g of carbs. Order a few pieces of grilled chicken is super simple and super quick. Just remember to skip most of the sides and ketchup, but if you must have one, order an individual serving of green beans which is only 2g net carbs. If you prefer a salad, order without dressing and it will only be around 2g of carbs

Taco Bell

You may be able to order just the side dishes, the chicken, beef, lettuce and guacamole come in cheap and the number of carbs is pretty decent also.

Gas stations

Many gas stations offer eggs, deli meat and string cheeses which can be a viable option, also if they sell a breakfast sandwich, just discard the bun and you will be left with tasty sausage, egg and cheese.

Wendy's

Their double stack order without a bun comes in at 4g carbs, it is also easy on the wallet, they also have the ultimate chicken grill sandwich which is 5g carbs without the bun.

In-N-Out Burger

If you are lucky to live close to these guys, they will supply a burger without a bun, but instead of a bun, they will supply it in a lettuce wrap. Just swap the house spread and replace it with mustard and extra pickles.

Chipotle

Fancy Mexican? For spicy food, this is probably your best bet, just order the burrito bowl without rice, or they have a wonderful salad available. The meat, cheese, sour cream, lettuce and salsa costs extra, but it can be worth the little extra to be satisfied with some wholesome food without any fear of overstepping your carb mark.

Unwich

All of their sandwiches can be ordered without bread or tortilla which is replaced by a lettuce wrap, as you can order online you are able to check your carbs as you go.

Five Guys Burger and Fries

These guys will supply your burger without a bun and without any hassle. They will supply a lettuce wrap or you can take it to go in an aluminum tray. You can also pick your toppings from their menu board. They also give extra cheese and extra bacon at no extra charge, if you find yourself dining in, they also have peanuts in the shell which you can nibble on while waiting for your burger.

Chapter 3 – What to Avoid

Before we start on what must be avoided, if you are a serious athletic person, your daily intake will be quite different to a normal person. Your exercise regime will have to be supported and your calorific intake will have to be adjusted accordingly.

Although protein is not to be avoided while on the keto diet, it will still have to be eaten in moderation, any high amount of protein can raise the body's insulin levels whilst at the same time, lowering your ketone levels. A safe estimation of protein that should be consumed in one day is around 35% of your maximum calorific intake for the day. It should also be noted, not all fats are equal, and any oils that are high in polyunsaturated fats (Omega-6) should be avoided such as soy, safflower, and cottonseed amongst others. Sources of these include, salad dressings and mayonnaise.

Foods to Avoid

Factory farmed meats and fish contain high amounts of Omega-6 and other chemicals which can be harmful to humans.

Liquid eggs these contain many additives and can be loaded with fructose corn syrup, this is a source of high carbs.

Artificial Sweeteners as a replacement for sugar they may be ok, but they can induce cravings and they have no health benefits at all.

Fresh milk should be consumed in moderation or avoided altogether, we are led to believe fresh milk is good for us, but as the majority has been pasteurized all the good bacteria has been killed off, another thing you may not realize is, milk actually has a high carb count, one cup contains about 12 grams of carbs. If you are drinking tea or coffee, try to use a bit of cream as an alternative.

Sweetened foods and drinks should be avoided

Legumes and beans are one of the staple vegetables in our diet, these should be avoided along with lentils, kidney beans, and chickpeas.

Fruits can contain high levels of carbs, grapes, tangerines, bananas, mango and pineapple should be avoided as with any dried fruits, all is not lost, if you crave fruit, small portions of berries are ok.

Starches and grains are in most of what we eat, and most of our current diet will consist of these in one form or another. The foods to avoid consist of rice, pasta, wheat based cereals, crackers, cookies, and Pizza.

Root vegetables are some of the main culprits, potatoes, carrots, and parsnips etc should all be avoided.

Condiments such as ketchup and sauces are highly processed and contain added sugars, unhealthy fats, and other additives, ketchup for instance contains 5 grams of carbs per tablespoon whereas honey mustard contains 11 grams of carbs per sachet.

Alcohol is made from grains and you guessed it, carbs are present in grains

Sauces – gravy or packet sauces contain flour or sugar, either choose low-carb versions or make your own

Yogurt – a normal container of Greek yogurt will contain 6 grams of carbs from natural sugars, flavored yogurts can contain up to 30 grams.

Coleslaw – 5% of the contents of coleslaw contains up to 14 grams of carbs.

Peanut Butter – 2 tablespoons of peanut butter contain 14 grams of carbs

Balsamic Oil – salad dressings can have varying amounts of carbs. Some fat free options can contain up to 12 grams per serving.

Fried Foods – chicken nuggets and chicken sandwiches from some of the more popular chains contain around 10 grams of carbs

And lastly, one that defies all logic, low fat or diet products like sugar-free diet foods, these are highly processed and contain high amounts of carbs. Low fat dressings etc, food manufacturers normally replace fats with sugars to maintain flavor, stay with full fat versions but limit your portion size

Chapter 4 – The Keto Advantage

Over the decades there has been much discussion about low carb diets. Since 2002 there have been over 20 human studies on diets of this sort, and it is a low carb diet that consistently comes out on top. I will now explain the top 10 advantages that have been found by following the Keto diet. It is not only weight loss that is affected, you will find an abundance of other health benefits it can bring to you.

Less Hungry

It is true, dieting makes you hungry. This is the main reason people end up miserable, and end up quitting whatever diet they are on. But with the keto diet, you automatically have a reduction in appetite. It is shown in the studies that, people who eat more fat and protein, end up eating fewer calories, so you will actually feel less hungry than on most other diets.

More Sustainable Weight Loss

Whilst these studies show you become less hungry, by following a low carb diet, they also came to the conclusion that you can lose more weight, and lose weight faster than people on low-fat diets. Even if the ones on a low-fat diet are restricting their calorific intake.

Over the first couple of weeks on the diet, the Keto diet will get rid of excess water from the body. Insulin levels become lower due to the restriction of carbohydrate intake, which allows the kidneys to start removing excess sodium, it is this that can help lead to a rapid weight loss on the first week or two.

It has also been shown, the amount of weight lost by following the Keto diet can be 2 or 3 times more than by following a low-fat diet, and all this without feeling hungry! Surely that is a major advantage?

More Fat is Lost from the Belly

Not all fat on the body is the same and it is the location of these fat deposits that dictate what disease you will be prone to, but unfortunately when on a diet, it is the body that decides where to take the fat from. Luckily, the Keto diet takes a greater proportion of fat from around the abdomen. The most important thing to know is we have fat under the skin, and then fat in the abdominal cavity which builds up around the internal organs.

This fat build up can increase inflammation, insulin resistance and is one of the major factors of metabolic dysfunction, which is most common in a western diet of today.

Luckily, the Keto diet is super-efficient at reducing these internal body fats first, this helps to reduce the risk of heart disease and type 2 diabetes. The amount of weight loss that any one person can lose will vary, although tests were conducted by the American Journal of Clinical Nutrition which showed, men who followed the ketogenic diet for a period of 4 weeks, lost an average of 12 pounds in weight. All the while they were able to eat a fewer number of calories without the hunger normally associated with regular diets.

Triglycerides (fat molecules) Reduce

You will be pleased to know, low-carb diets are very effective at lowering the levels of triglycerides in the blood. These fat molecules are what increase the risk of heart disease.

The main cause for these levels to increase is carbohydrate consumption. So as these are dramatically reduced, the levels in the blood of these triglycerides are also reduced. It should also be noted, people who actually follow a low-fat diet compared to the Keto diet can have an increase in triglyceride levels.

Increased HDL levels

HDL (High-Density Lipoprotein) is many times referred to as the good cholesterol, and it is HDL that carries cholesterol away from the body to the liver where it gets flushed from the system or re-used. It is also known that if you have higher levels of HDL, you are less prone to the risk of heart disease. Another indicator that can show if a person is prone to heart disease, is the Triglycerides to HDL ratio. The higher it is, the greater the risk. This is another way the Keto diet excels. This ratio can see a much greater improvement as HDL levels are raised whilst triglyceride levels are lowered.

Lowered LDL levels

LDL is the opposite to HDL, and is referred to as the bad cholesterol. It is this one, that leads to heart disease if the levels are high in the body. Studies have also shown the size of the LDL particles is also an important factor, small particles give the greatest risk whereas larger particles give a lower risk. Once again, the Keto diet helps with this. By being a low carb diet, the particles of LDL change from small to large, thus reducing the number that can float around the body.

Blood Sugar and Insulin Levels

When carbs are consumed, the body breaks these down and they get converted into simple sugars, namely glucose, by the digestive system. It is these simple sugars upon entering the blood stream that raise the body's blood sugar levels. To combat and maintain these levels the body produces the hormone insulin.

In normal people, this increased amount of insulin is not much of a problem, but in people that have insulin resistance, it is a major problem and can lead to type 2 diabetes and figures for people with this problem are currently over 300 million worldwide.

The keto diet can provide you with the solution to this, by reducing carb intake, the body does not have to produce as much insulin, as the blood sugar levels from a reduction in carbs is greatly reduced.

Studies have also shown, by following the Keto diet, diabetics can actually reduce the need for medication within 6 months.

It should be noted, if you are currently on medication, you should consult your doctor before proceeding.

Lowered Blood Pressure

High blood pressure (Hypertension) can be the root of many illnesses in humans. These can include kidney failure, strokes and heart disease to name but a few. The Keto diet is a very effective way of reducing blood pressure which can lower the risk of these illnesses.

Metabolic Syndrome

Metabolic Syndrome is a collection of symptoms that can lead to diabetes and heart disease. These symptoms range from Abdominal obesity, high blood sugar levels low HDL levels and High triglycerides, although these can be serious they can all be reduced by following the keto diet.

Brain Functions

Originally the Keto diet was introduced to help treat children who suffered from epilepsy. This was something, it had many successful results in doing. Over 50 % of children treated showed a 50% reduction in seizures while 16 % of the children actually stopped having seizures completely.

Some parts of the brain can only burn glucose, as the carb intake is reduced on the keto diet. The liver converts protein to glucose, which can supply these parts of the brain. The other parts of the brain are powered by ketones. These are produced when the body is starved of carbs. This is the main reason; the Keto diet is so successful at treating epilepsy. Not only that, more recent studies have shown the diet can be helpful in other forms of brain disorder, namely Alzheimer's disease and Parkinson's Disease.

Cancer

Research has shown sugar is the main fuel which can feed cancer cells, the cancer cells ferment the sugars to produce oxygen, this, in turn, increases the amount of inflammation in the body. This was discovered by Dr.Otto Warburg in the 1930's. He also found, when the body has a low blood sugar content, the amount of inflammation is reduced and the cancer cells are unable to thrive as the blood is fully oxygenated naturally.

Diet Comparisons

5:2 Diet

This diet is, you eat for 5 days of the week and then fast on the two remaining days. Fans of this diet, claim it can help lose weight, make you live longer and help against Alzheimer's and dementia. Although fasting for 2 days per week is too daunting for most people.

Dukan Diet

This diet is based on low carbs and a high protein intake. There are 4 stages, stage one is a strict lean protein diet for 5 days. Here carbs are off limits apart from a small portion of oat bran. Phases 2,3 and 4 introduce fruits, vegetables, and carbs. For long-term sustainability, it is classed as unhealthy, as there is no balance in the nutrition.

Paleo Diet

This one is also known as the "caveman" diet. Foods that can be hunted, fished or gathered can be eaten. Anything that is refined or processed is strictly off-limits, thus the diet lacks food variety. So, it easy to get bored with it quickly and quit.

South Beach Diet

Originally for American heart patients, it has no calorie counting and no portion limits. It encourages you to eat 3 meals a day along with 2 snacks and the addition of a healthy exercise plan. Overall it is reducing the GI (glycemic index) foods, altogether there are 2 phases, but phase 1 may be too restrictive for adults with a normal lifestyle. The way the diet works, any weight loss will consist of water and carbs, not only fat. Once you return to normal eating habits, these will be replaced quickly.

Chapter 5 – Essential Groceries

Whilst on the keto diet, your shopping habits will change, as will most of the contents you have in your kitchen and pantry. The list below, is by no means complete. The aim is to give you a good starting point for what items you should be considering to stock., and what is available and what you should be avoiding.

The best advice is to eat a variety of fresh meat, wild caught seafood, plenty of fresh vegetables and natural fats which have not been processed. If used in moderation, some canned goods can be used as long as they are not processed meals.

Most of the items below are items that should be in stock in your kitchen, In the recipe sections of the book, I will give specifics of what ingredients you will need for the recipes.

Pantry Items

Dried Smoked Meat sticks – Beef jerky

Pork Rinds – use these as an alternative to breadcrumbs, or sprinkle on salads and soups to add flavor.

Sugar-Free Salad Dressings and most bottled Hot Sauces

Canned Tomatoes – check carb and added sugar levels

Pasta or pizza sauce – check for added thickeners or added sugars

Canned Fish and seafood's - Tuna, Shrimp, Sardines, Crab, and Anchovies.

Chicken or Vegetable stock, Apple Cider and Wine Vinegar

Nut Butter – they must be natural and unsweetened

Low Carbohydrate Vegetables - green beans, sauerkraut, and okra (with no added sugar)

Lemon or lime juice – contains 1 gram of carbs per spoonful

Horseradish

Salsa's – check ingredients to find one that is suitable with no added sugars

Pickles which contain no added sugar

Natural mustard – no added sugar

Capers

Cooking and Baking Ingredients

Nut Flours (Almond Flour etc) or flour substitutes

Cooking Oil - Coconut Oil and Peanut Oil are suitable

Unsweetened Extracts - Almond, Vanilla and Lemon etc

Whey Protein Powder - Chocolate, Plain, and Vanilla (don't forget daily protein levels)

Unsweetened Cocoa Powder

Herbs & Spices

Herbs and spices are one way in which you can transform the taste of your meals, although check contents to make sure contain no sweeteners or MSG

Black & White Pepper and Sea Salt

Chili Powder & Cayenne Pepper, Curry Powder & Garam Masala

Cumin & Oregano, Rosemary & Thyme, Nutmeg, Cloves & Ginger

Nuts & Seeds

Although these are on your shopping list, you should be aware they contain Omega 6 fatty acids, so they should be eaten in moderation, as they are so small, it does not take many to increase your carbohydrate intake.

Seeds (Sesame, Sunflower, and Pumpkin)

Nuts (Walnuts, Pecans, Hazelnut, Almond & Coconut)

Peanuts are classed as a legume so should be avoided.

Vegetables

With vegetables, it is best to try to stick to green leafy veggies and avoid any root vegetables.

Seaweeds any type of sea vegetables are suitable.

Peppers and Capsicum

Broccoli, Cabbage

Cucumber, Lettuce, green leafy vegetables like kale, spinach & watercress

Shallots

Zucchini

Fermented vegetables can also be used, the most common are Kimchi and Sauerkraut

Meats

When you buy meats, these should be grass fed and organic. The use of pesticides or antibiotics will not have been used on these animals.

All meats following the above advice are good to eat. The only limiting factor is your daily limits. In this way the transition to ketosis will not be affected.

Pork all cuts of pork can be used (chops, steaks, ribs & roast)

Beef all cuts of beef can be used (roast, ribs & steaks)

Lamb, Mutton & Goat

Wild Game

Venison

Bacon, Hams & Sausages (Carb count for any of these should be less than 1 gram per serving

Another category in the meats section is organ meats. Although not popular with a lot of people, they are one of the most nutritious foods available. The following organs can be eaten from almost any animal

Heart, Liver, Kidney, Tongue & Tripe

Seafood & Shellfish

Fish or seafood should be preferred over poultry and meats if it has not been farmed and manmade feeds have been used. Fish and seafood's can be in any form either Fresh or Frozen.

Shellfish, although normally a little more expensive, can be worth the little cost as the nutrients gained from it is much higher than meats and poultry

Bass & Cod, Haddock & Halibut, Herring & Mackerel, Tuna, Tilapia, Trout & Salmon, Shrimp, Scallops, Prawns and Lobster, Clams, Mussels, Oysters, Caviar

Canned fish that is packed with oils or brine and not in sauce e.g. tuna, sardines & salmon

Delicatessen Meat

In an emergency, these give you better options to other alternatives, which contain high levels of carbohydrates, as with any foods that have been prepared check the ingredients for any added sugars or sweeteners.

Salami, Pepperoni, Prosciutto, Cold cuts (Turkey & Pastrami)

Poultry

With poultry or any other fowl, the best option is to find ones that are organically raised.

Chicken, Turkey, Duck and others.

Dairy Products

Eggs

Greek Yoghurt, this should be plain and full fat with a carb count less than 7g per individual serving

Heavy Creams & Sour Cream, Cream Cheese, and Soft Cheeses

Hard Cheese like Cheddar & Parmesan

Fruits

A lot of fruits should be avoided in large quantities. Some fruits consumed in moderation will be ok. Berries which are in season are preferred: Raspberry, Strawberry, Blackberry, Blueberries & Cranberry all have a low sugar content and are full of antioxidants

Avocados can be used as a snack or made into guacamole for dipping

Olives, Lemon & Lime

Legumes

Most legumes should be avoided, although in small quantities peas and green beans are ok.

Fats & Oils

As was mentioned, the Keto diet is high in fat and low carbs, so fats and oils play a big part as they make up a majority of the bodies calorific intake. All you must be aware of is the fats you are taking are healthy fats.

Olive Oils, Avocado Oils, Coconut Oils, Palm Shortening, Duck Fat, Sesame Oils, Cocoa Butter

Butter, if you can tolerate dairy products.

Drinks

As with most drinks, it is better to check the ingredients for any hidden sugars they may contain.

Coconut Milk & Almond Milk

Tea both normal & Herbal, Coffee

Sparkling Mineral Water & Club Soda and normal water

Chapter 6 – 5 Day Recipe Guide

The Keto diet has a few side effects that may happen in the first 5 days. These are normal, as with any diet and will quickly pass after a couple of days. There will also be a difference if the diet is for children or adults. Most of these side effects are manageable, if you understand why they happen. To have this knowledge beforehand means you will be able to minimize the effects and are less likely to quit.

It only takes a short time for your body to enter a state of ketosis; from this point, the side effects will subside as your body adapts to burning fat for energy rather than glucose.

Please always, always seek medical advice before you start. Prioritize your health for safety, and long term longevity.

Low Blood Sugar (Hypoglycemia)

As your body is used to a high carb diet, it creates insulin to counteract the sugar that gets created from your carbohydrate intake. Once your carb quantity drops on the Keto diet, you may experience low blood sugar episodes. Symptoms include, Confusion, Dizziness, Feeling shaky, Hunger, Headaches, Irritability, Pounding heart; racing pulse, Pale skin, Sweating, Trembling, Weakness, Anxiety. It can seem scary if you have not experienced it before. The easiest way to maintain this is by glucose tablets, so when you feel this is about to happen, take one or two tablets and this should be enough to prevent this happening.

Headaches

Any major change in diet can cause headaches for no apparent reason. You may become light-headed, and also have flu-like symptoms which can occur over several days. These headaches happen as there is a mineral imbalance due to diet changes. The best way to resolve this quickly is to add one-quarter of a teaspoon of salt into a glass of water and drink. You should then sit down for 15 – 20 minutes for the effects to take place. To prevent this happening you should drink plenty of water and increase your salt intake for the first few days. This can effectively stop the chance of headaches.

Fatigue and Dizziness

Your body will start to lose stored water content, so it is crucial this is replaced, as a result, there will be many minerals you will lose over the first week on the diet. With low minerals, you may feel tired, dizzy and lightheaded along with the chance of getting unwanted muscle cramps - and a possibility of itchy skin. To combat these effects, increase the amount of green leafy vegetables you consume. Or as a backup, it is possible to use multivitamin tablets that provide the recommended daily allowance for the lost minerals that you require. Stay clear of any vegetables that are high in carbs, as discussed earlier.

Constipation

This is one of the most common side effects. This comes from losing fluids and becoming dehydrated, loss of salt, a magnesium deficiency or too many dairy/nut products. If things don't change by taking vitamin tablets (to improve your magnesium intake), you may have to reduce your dairy product intake even more.

Diarrhea

These symptoms normally only last for a few days, thankfully. Once you have increased your fat content, your body should adjust and these symptoms should subside. Always drink lots of water to replace the lost fluids so as not to become dehydrated.

Interrupted Sleep Patterns

Some people mention they have problems sleeping whilst on the Keto diet - if this happens it can be a sign your insulin levels are low. To solve this, have a small snack that contains an equal amount of protein and carbs just before going to bed. This will help balance your insulin level for the night. Just for the short term.

Heart Palpitations

This can happen to some people, and not happen to others, like if you drink a strong cup of coffee. Although whilst on the Keto diet, it can be a sign a person has low blood pressure. Always seek medical advice if you are not sure.

Sugar Cravings

This is one of the most difficult side effects to resist. Just give yourself time and these will subside in anything from a few days up to a period of around 21 days. Several ways to combat these cravings is doing some light exercise or finding something that can occupy your mind. Sugar cravings will only last for an hour; so, this will have gone by the time you have completed your exercise. You can also have a snack consisting of a few ounces of protein, either in the form of a small salad or a small, quick to prepare smoothie.

This is just a few of the most common side effects although some people report they have suffered from the following:

Hair loss – this is not linked to the Keto diet directly, it is just a complete change in diet that can cause this in some people.

Low Thyroid T3 Hormone levels – this can always happen in reduced calorie diets; it is an effect of the body's reduced calorific intake.

If the Keto diet is followed for long periods, there are several other side effects that may arise and which can affect children more than adults.

Kidney Stones –children can be affected more commonly than adults; estimates say there is a 5% possibility a child can get kidney stones after following the diet.

Stunted Growth – this would be a problem for children, there can be a reduced amount of growth factor 1 hormone being produced. With stunted growth, there can be a risk of bone fractures.

Again, a child should NEVER be placed on a ketogenic diet, the consequences are very drastic and harmful while children are still growing, it is better to give them all the fruits, vegetables, carbs, and proteins, in a balanced diet, and limit their processed sugar found in candy, sodas, and sweets.

Stage 1 - The First 5 Days

So now that you know what to expect, you're ready with Stage 1 of this diet.

The recipes in your Stage 1 diet are designed to be as low on carbs as possible (limiting it to no more than around 20 grams per day), so that you will deplete your glycogen stores and reach a state of ketosis quickly. This can happen as fast as 48 hours so 5 days should guarantee you'll get there.

We "lighten up" on the carb intake in Stage 2 so that your food options become less restrictive.

A shopping list is at the end of this chapter to help you in your preparation for the Stage 1 diet.

Day 1 - Breakfast

Fried Eggs & Tomatoes - Serves 1

Prep time 10 min, Cook time 10 min

Nutrition per serving: Calories 115, Fat 16g, Protein, 16g, Carbs 8g

Ingredients

1 large tomato halved

1 teaspoon of olive oil

Salt & pepper to taste

2 eggs

1 scallion finely sliced

½ tablespoon of parmesan cheese

Instructions

Heat the broiler to 180C,

Drizzle oil on the face of tomato and sprinkle with salt, pepper, and a little parmesan, place cut side up under the broiler. Cook for 3 – 4 minutes until soft, while these are cooking,

Heat remaining oil in a medium skillet over medium heat, break the eggs and place into the skillet, cover and cook until your desired liking.

Transfer eggs and tomatoes to serving plate, sprinkle with remaining parmesan, scallions, salt and pepper to taste.

Day 1 - Lunch

Stuffed Bacon Burgers - Serves 2

Prep time 10 minutes, cook time 15 minutes

Nutrition per serving: Calories 177, Fat 10g, Protein 17g, 3g carbs

Ingredients

2 slices bacon

1/8 cup onion, chopped

1/4 can mushroom pieces, drained and finely chopped

100g lean ground beef

60g pork sausage

1 tablespoon Parmesan cheese, grated

1 pinch teaspoon pepper

1 pinch garlic powder

1 tablespoon steak sauce

Instructions

Heat skillet over medium heat, add bacon and cook until crispy, remove all but two tablespoons of the dripping, add onion to the pan with dripping and cook until tender.

Crumble the cold bacon and return to the skillet with the mushrooms and place on one side.

Combine ground beef, pork sausage, cheese, pepper, garlic powder and steak sauce in a medium bowl.

Once mixed form into 4 patties, divide bacon and onion mixture and place onto two of the patties, put the other two patties on top and press down to seal the edges.

Grill over medium coals or under the broiler until well done.

Note: sausage in burgers requires thorough cooking.

Day 1 - Dinner

Goat Cheese Frittata with Spinach - Serves 2

Prep time 15 minutes, cook time 20 minutes

Nutrition per serving: Calories 399, Fat 31g, Protein 23g, Carbs 9g

Ingredients

2 tablespoons olive oil

½ medium onion, sliced thinly

Salt & pepper to taste

3 cups baby spinach

5 large eggs, beaten

1/2 cup goats cheese, crumbled

1 tablespoon white wine vinegar

3 cups mixed greens

Instructions

Heat oven to 180C

Heat 1 tablespoon of the oil in a medium ovenproof nonstick skillet over medium-high heat.

Add the onion and a pinch of salt and pepper, cook while stirring occasionally, until tender, 3 to 4 minutes.

Add the spinach, cook while tossing, until wilted, 1 to 2 minutes.

Add the beaten eggs and sprinkle with goat's cheese.

Cook until the mixture starts to set around the edges, around 1 to 2 minutes.

Transfer to the oven and bake until set, 10 to 12 minutes.

Mix together the vinegar, 2 tablespoons of oil, and a pinch of salt and pepper in a large bowl. Add the greens and toss to cover the greens with the mixture.

Serve with the frittata and bread

Day 2- Breakfast

Scrambled Eggs with Cheese - Serves 1

Nutrition per serving: 453 Calories, Fat43g, Protein 19g, Carbs 1.2g

Ingredients

2 Large Eggs

2 Tablespoon Butter

¼ cup Cheddar Cheese

Instructions

Heat a pan on medium heat, add the butter.

Once the butter has melted, add the 2 beaten eggs

Cook the eggs slowly stirring occasionally

Add cheese and mix gently until combined

Transfer to a serving plate

Day 2 - Lunch

Simple Lunch Salad with Tuna – serves 1

Nutrition Per Serving: 624 Calories, Fat 63.9g, Protein 10.8g, Carbs 1.2g,

Ingredients

1 can of tuna in brine

2 tablespoon of Olive Oil

2 Cups Spinach

1 tablespoon of Parmesan Cheese grated

1 ½ teaspoon of Dijon Mustard

¼ Lemon zest

Meat Specified in Day-by-Day

Instructions

In a small bowl combine all wet ingredients

In another bowl combine meat and spinach

Pour wet ingredients over meat and spinach when ready to eat.

Day 2 - Dinner

Stir fried beef with orange -serves 1

Prep time 20 minutes, cook time 20 minutes

Nutrition per serving: Calories 649, Fat 44.5g, Protein 53.5, Carbs 1.9g

Ingredients

100g Beefsteak thinly sliced

1/4 cup Beef Broth

1 tablespoon of Coconut Oil

1/2 Medium onion diced

Zest and juice of 1/4 Orange

2 cloves garlic minced

1 inch sliced ginger

1 pinch ground cinnamon

½ teaspoon Soy Sauce

½ teaspoon Fish Sauce

1 Bay Leaf

Instructions

Dice your vegetables and cut beef into 1" thin slices

Heat coconut oil in a cast iron skillet over medium heat and add diced onion, garlic, and ginger.

Cook for 1 minute then add beef and cook for 5 minutes, add soy sauce and fish sauce, bay leaf, cinnamon and orange juice and beef broth.

Raise heat and cook until juices have started to thicken.

Transfer to serving plate and sprinkle with orange zest.

Day 3 - Breakfast

Herbed Eggs - serves 1

Prep time 10 minutes Cooking time 10 minutes

Nutrition per serving: Calories 710, Fat 63g, Protein 30.1g, Carbs 3.3g

Ingredients

1/2 tablespoon unsalted butter

2 eggs

1 tablespoon milk

Salt and black pepper

1/4 cup chopped mixed fresh herbs

1 scallions chopped finely

Instructions

Heat butter in a large nonstick skillet over medium heat.

In a medium bowl beat the eggs, milk and add 1 pinch of salt and pepper

Pour into the pan and stir occasionally or cooked to liking 5 minutes approx.

Fold in herbs and scallions and then transfer to a serving plate

Day 3 - Lunch

Chicken and Mushroom Soup: serves 2

Prep time 10 minutes Cooking time 10 minutes

Nutrition per serving: Calories 385, Fat 33g, Protein 30.1g, Carbs 7.2g

Ingredients

250g boneless chicken breast

2 cups chicken stock

1 cup fresh mushrooms, quartered

4 tablespoons sesame oil

2 tablespoons Sherry

2 tablespoons fresh parsley, chopped

Instructions

Slice the chicken breast into thin slices

In a medium saucepan add the chicken stock and bring to a boil, when starting to boil add the chicken and mushrooms.

When the soup begins to boil again, remove from the heat add the sesame oil and sherry then taste for seasoning, add salt and pepper as necessary

Serve in individual soup bowls, and sprinkle with parsley.

Day 3 - Dinner

Chicken and Bacon Sausage Stir Fry Serves 1 plus 2 leftover portions

Nutrition per serving: Calories 451, Fat 28.3g, Protein 35.7g, Carbs 7.3g

Ingredients

4 Chicken Sausages

3 Cups Broccoli Florets

3 Cups Spinach

1/2 Cup Parmesan Cheese grated

1/2 Cup Tomato Sauce

1/4 Cup Red Wine

2 tablespoon of Salted Butter

2 cloves of garlic minced. Minced Garlic

½ a teaspoon of red pepper flakes

Instructions

Slice the 4 chicken sausages into ¼ pieces

In a medium saucepan boil half a pan of water and then add the broccoli florets cook for 5 minutes

In a skillet, cook the sausage pieces until golden on all sides

Push the sausage pieces to the side and then add the butter, add the garlic to the butter and sauté for 1 minute, combine everything together and add the hot broccoli, pour in the red pepper flakes and the tomato sauce along with the red wine.

Move your sausages to one side of the pan, then add the butter.

Put your garlic in the butter and let it sauté for 1 minute.

Mix everything together and then adds your broccoli.

Pour in the tomato sauce, red wine, and add red pepper flakes.

Combine everything together and cook until it is ready.

Mix together, add your spinach with salt and pepper and let it cook down.

Simmer this for 5-10 minutes.

Day 4 - Breakfast

Ham and eggs with Cheddar and chives: Serves 2

Preparation time: 10 minutes, cooking time 10 minutes

Nutrition Per Serving: Calories 369.36, Fat 26.74g, Protein 28.69g, Carbs 2.21g

Ingredients

1 tablespoons unsalted butter

4 eggs

2 tablespoons milk or water

½ teaspoon salt

¼ teaspoon freshly ground black pepper

1 cup diced cooked ham

1 cup shredded sharp Cheddar

1/4 cup chopped fresh chives

Instructions

Heat a skillet over medium heat and melt the butter.

Add the ham and sauté until browned.

Meanwhile, in a large bowl, beat together the eggs, milk, 1/2 teaspoon salt, and 1/4 teaspoon pepper. Pour into the pan and cook, and stir occasionally, to your desired taste approx. 4 to 5 minutes

Add grated cheddar and chives just before the eggs begin to set.

Day 4 - Lunch

Greek Frittata - Serves 2

Preparation Time 10 minutes, Cooking time 25- 30 minutes

Nutrition Per Serving: Calories 461, Fat 35g, Protein 26g, Carbs 8g

Ingredients

1 1/2 tablespoons olive oil

5 large eggs

Pinch of salt and pepper

10-ounce baby spinach

2 cups grape tomatoes halved

2 scallions thinly sliced

4 ounces' feta cheese crumbled

Instructions

Pre-Heat oven to 350° F.

Add the oil to a 2-quart casserole and place in the oven for 5 minutes.

In a medium bowl, beat the eggs, salt, pepper then add the tomatoes, spinach, and scallions, mix until combined and then add the crumbled feta cheese

Remove the casserole dish from oven, pour in the egg mixture and bake until the frittata is brown around the edges and a knife comes out clean from the center. 20 – 30 minutes

Day 4 - Dinner

Salmon with Avocado & Lime– Serves 2

Prep Time 20 minutes Cooking time 15 minutes

Nutrition Per Serving: Calories 420, Fat 27g, Protein 37g, Carbs 5g

Ingredients

2 x 6 oz. salmon fillets

1 large avocado

1/2 lime juice and zest

2 tablespoon of red onion (diced)

100 g cauliflower

1 tablespoon of olive oil

Pinch of salt and pepper to taste

Instructions

Add cauliflower to blender and pulse until the size is similar to rice

Heat a small skillet over medium heat, add cauliflower and cook covered until done about 8 minutes

Add salt and pepper to taste

In a food processor add the flesh of the avocado with the juice of ½ lime along with the red onion blend on high until you have a creamy consistency.

Heat a skillet over medium-high heat add 1 tablespoon of olive oil

Season salmon with salt and pepper then place skin side down

Cook for 5 minutes then turn and cook for another 4 or 5 minutes or until done

Divide cauliflower between serving plates, add salmon and cover with the avocado lime dressing

Sprinkle with a little lime zest.

Day 5 - Breakfast

Blender Pancakes – Serves 1

Preparation Time 5 minutes, Cooking time 10 minutes

Nutrition Per Serving: Calories 450, Fat 29g, Protein 41g, Carbs 4g

Ingredients

2 large eggs

1 scoop Protein Powder plain or vanilla flavor

1 good pinch of cinnamon

2 oz. cream cheese

1 pinch salt

Instructions

Add the cream cheese, eggs, protein powder, cinnamon and salt into a blender

Blend for about 10 seconds until mixed and then let it sit.

Heat a small skillet over medium heat

Pour out about 1/4 of the batter slowly into the pan.

Cook until small bubbles start to appear on the surface, slide spatula underneath and turn

Cook the other side of the pancake until starting to turn golden brown

Serve with syrup or butter, but be aware of your calorie intake.

Day 5 - Lunch

Garlic Cauliflower– Serves 2

Preparation Time 10 minutes, Cooking time 15 minutes

Nutrition Per Serving: Calories 60, Fat 6g, Protein 4g, Carbs 3g

Ingredients

2 cups cauliflower

1 tablespoon toasted sesame seeds

1 tablespoon virgin olive oil

Dash of paprika for coating

2 large cloves garlic, minced

Pepper, to taste

Instructions

Half fill a medium sized saucepan with water and bring to the boil

Add the trimmed cauliflower florets and cook for around 2 minutes then drain

Heat a medium sized skillet over medium heat, add oil and garlic, cook until garlic starts to brown.

Add the cauliflower and stir-fry for 1 -2 minutes, add sesame seeds and toss to coat

Place of serving plates and sprinkle with paprika and pepper.

Day 5 - Dinner

Cheats Pasta with Cheesy Tomato Sauce– Serves 2

Preparation Time 15 minutes, Cooking time 15 minutes

Nutrition Per Serving: Calories 260, Fat 21g, Protein 12g, Carbs 5g

Ingredients

3 medium yellow or butternut squash

200 g streaky bacon

2 cloves garlic minced

1 big pinch of red pepper flakes

1 cup tomato sauce (regular can of sauce)

Sea Salt and black pepper to taste

1/4 cup Parmesan cheese grated

Instructions

In a medium skillet heat a small amount of oil on medium heat

Add bacon and cook until becoming crispy, remove bacon and cut into pieces once done

In the same pan add garlic and cook in bacon fat until starting to brown add red pepper flakes to combine flavors

To the pan add your tomato sauce, simmer until beginning to bubble then add bacon pieces

Spiralize the squash into noodle size of choice, add to the sauce and cook for 2 – 3 minutes until soft

Season with salt and pepper

Transfer to serving plates and cover with freshly grated parmesan

Week 1 Snacks

Pesto Crackers – 6 servings

Prep time 10 minutes, cook time 20 minutes

Nutrition per serving: Calories 210, Fat 19.3g, Protein 5g, Carbs 6g

Ingredients

1 ¼ cup Almond Flour

¼ tsp ground black pepper

½ tsp salt

½ tsp baking powder

¼ tsp dried basil

Pinch of cayenne pepper

1 clove garlic minced

2 tablespoon basil pesto

3 tablespoon Butter

Instructions

Preheat Oven to 160C

In a medium, Bowl adds Almond Flour, pepper, salt and baking powder, whisk until smooth.

Add Basil, Cayenne pepper, Garlic and stir until evenly combined

Add in the Pesto and whisk until the dough forms into coarse crumbs.

Slice the butter into the cracker mixture, mix with the fork or your fingers until the dough forms into a ball.

Transfer the dough to a prepared cookie sheet and spread out the dough thinly until it is about 1 ½ mm thick. Ensure equal thickness so the crackers will cook evenly

Bake for 14 to 17 minutes until the color will be Golden Brown.

Remove from the Oven once it is cooked, and slice into desired sizes

Keto Lava Cake – Serves 1

Prep time 10 minutes, cook time 15 minutes

Nutrition per serving: Calories 173, Fat 13g, Protein 8g, Carbs 4g

Ingredients

2 tablespoon cocoa powder

1-2 tablespoon powdered sweetener

1 medium egg

1 tablespoon heavy cream

½ teaspoon vanilla extract

1/4 teaspoon baking powder

Instructions

Preheat your oven to 190C.

In a small bowl mix the cocoa powder, powdered sweetener, baking soda and salt

In a small bowl, beat your egg until a little fluffy. The air in the egg is needed as there is no flour.

Wet a large mug with a little oil, and fill with cake batter, place on baking tray and bake for 10 – 15 minutes, the top of the cake should be firm but jiggly

You can also microwave your mug cake for about a minute. All microwaves are different, so once the minute is up, check up on your cake and if it's still not solid but jiggly on top, put it back in for 10-second intervals until done.

Mexican Fudge – 4 servings

Prep time 10 minutes, cook time 15 minutes

Nutrition per serving: Calories 629, Fat 53g, Protein 36g, Carbs 3g

Ingredients

4 eggs

8 ounces Monterey Jack cheese grated

8 ounces Cheddar cheese grated

1 can green chili, chopped finely

1 cup heavy cream

Instructions

Preheat oven to 180C

Grease an 8-inch square baking dish

Spread Monterey Jack cheese on the bottom of the dish and cover with chopped chilies

Cover with grated Cheddar cheese

In a small bowl whisk the eggs and the heavy cream and pour over the cheese

Bake for 30 minutes or until eggs are cooked and cheese it going golden

Cut into 2–inch squares, and serve warm.

Spiced Almonds – 16 servings

Prep time 10 minutes, cook time 30 minutes

Nutrition per serving: Calories 139, Fat 12g, Protein 5g, Carbs 6g

Ingredients

1 egg white

2 tablespoons water

4 cups almonds

3/4 cup powdered sweetener

1/2 teaspoon ground cloves

1/4 teaspoon ground nutmeg

1 1/4 teaspoons ground cinnamon

Instructions

Preheat oven to 120C

Whisk egg whites with water. Add nuts and stir until moist then drain.

In a small bowl combine dry ingredients, mixing well. Add nuts and toss until coated.

Spread nuts on lightly greased baking sheet. Bake for 25 to 30 minutes, toss occasionally. Cool completely before storing in airtight container

Strawberry Shake – Serves 1

Prep time 10 minutes,

Nutrition per serving: Calories 279, Fat 22g, Protein 14g, Carbs 7g

Ingredients

1/2 cup heavy cream

2 packets powdered sweetener or honey

1/2 cup frozen strawberries

1/4 cup water

5 ice cubes

Instructions

Add all ingredients to a blender

Blend on high until you have a smooth consistency

Day 1 to 5 Shopping list

Almond flour – 300g, Almonds – 1kg, Avocado – 1pc, Baby spinach – 1 pack

Bacon – 250g, baking powder – 50g, Basil pesto – 1 pack, Bay leaf – 1 pack,

Beef broth – 250ml, Beef steak – 100g, Boneless chicken breast – 250g,

Broccoli florets – 1 pack, Butter – 1 stick, Butternut squash – 3pcs,

Can of mushroom pieces – 250g, Canned tuna – 1 can, Cauliflower – 250g,

Cayenne pepper – 1 pack, Cheddar cheese – 250g, Chicken sausages – 4 pcs,

Chicken stock – 500ml, Cinnamon powder – 1 pack, Cloves – 1 pack,

Cocoa powder – 1 small pack, Coconut oil – 10ml, Cooked ham – 250g,

Cream cheese – 2oz, Dijon mustard – 1 jar, Dried basil – 1 small pack,

Eggs - 28, Fish sauce – 1 small bottle, Fresh chives – 1 small bunch,

Fresh parsley – 1 small bunch, Frozen berries – 200g, Feta cheese – 1 small pack,

Garlic – 2 whole garlic, Garlic powder – 1 small jar, Ginger 1 pc, Goats cheese – 50g,

Grape tomatoes – 350g, Green chili – 1 can, Ground beef – 100g,

Heavy cream – 370ml, Honey – 1 jar, Lemons – 1 pc,

Lime – 1 pc, Milk – 1 pint, Mixed greens – 1 pack, Mixed herbs – 1 jar

Monterrey Jack cheese – 8 oz, Nutmeg – 1 jar, Olive oil – 250 ml,

Oranges – 1pc, Paprika – 1 small pack, Parmesan cheese – 4 g, Pork sausage – 60g

Powdered sweetener – 1 small pack, Protein powder – 1 pack, Red onions – 4pcs,

Red pepper flakes – 1 small pack, Red wine – 1 bottle, Salmon fillets – 12oz

Salt and pepper 1 small pack of each, Scallions or spring onions – 1 bunch

Sesame oil – 1 small bottle, Sesame seeds – 1 small pack, Sherry – 1 small bottle,

Soy sauce – 1 small bottle, Spinach – 1 large pack

Steak sauce – 1 small bottle, Tomato sauce – 1ltr, Tomatoes – 300g, Vanilla extract – 1 small bottle, White wine vinegar – 1 small bottle

Chapter 7 – Week 2 Days 6 - 12

Stage 2 - The Next 2 Weeks

Congratulations! You've made it through Stage 1's first 5 days. You'll find that the recipes for the next 2 weeks is perhaps a little more balanced in the macros. Have fun with it. Follow the recipes as is or mix and match, if you like. Make the ones you like again and skip the ones you don't.

Day 6 - Breakfast

Mini Crust Less Quiches: Serves 3 (12 individual quiches)

Prep time 15 minutes, cook time 25 minutes

Nutrition per serving Calories: 382, Fat 28g, Protein 22g, Carbs 5.3g (based on 4)

Ingredients

14 large eggs

3 plum tomatoes, diced

⅔ cup mozzarella cheese torn into small pieces

⅓ cup cheddar cheese grated

⅓ cup white onion finely diced

⅓ cup sliced pickled jalapenos

⅔ cup salami diced

⅓ cup heavy cream

Instructions

Preheat the oven to 160C and grease a 15" x 11" muffin tin.

In a large bowl add all of the ingredients and mix well, season with salt and pepper

Divide the batter into the muffin tin equally and bake for about 25 minutes.

Can be stored in the refrigerator and reheated

Day 6 - Lunch

Ham & Cheddar Wraps – Serves 1

Prep time 10 minutes, Cooking time 10 minutes

Nutrition per serving: Calories: 600, Fat 44g, Protein 27g, Carbs 8g

Ingredients

1 low carb wrap

2 tablespoon mayonnaise

2 oz cheddar grated

2 oz sliced ham

Pickles or jalapenos to taste thinly sliced

Salt, pepper to taste

Instructions

Heat skillet on medium heat, place wrap in skillet and warm for 30 seconds

On the warm wrap, spread the mayonnaise

Place ham slices and then sprinkle with grated cheese

Add sliced pickle or jalapenos according to taste

Fold ends inwards and roll tightly

Day 6 - Dinner

Chicken Quesadilla – Serves 1

Preparation time: 15 minutes, cooking time 15 minutes

Calories : 654, Fat 43g, Protein 52g, Carbs 7g

Ingredients

1 tablespoon of olive oil

1 low carb wrap

3 oz. cheddar cheese grated

2.5 oz. chicken breast thinly sliced

½ avocado, sliced thinly

1 teaspoon chopped jalapeño

¼ teaspoon salt

Instructions

In a small skillet, add a small amount of oil and cook the chicken strips thoroughly

Place the wrap on a frying pan wide enough to allow the wrap to lay as fully flat as possible on a medium heat.

After 2 minutes, flip the wrap over and begin laying the grated cheddar cheese. Don't get too close to the edges, leave an inch space

Add the chicken breast pieces, avocado and jalapeño to one half of the wrap.

Fold the wrap over with a spatula and press down to flatten, the cheese will stick the quesadilla together.

Take off the pan and cut into thirds.

Day 7 - Breakfast

Chocolate and Peanut Butter Muffins (6 muffins)

Preparation time 15 minutes, cooking time 15 minutes

Nutrition per serving: Calories 530, Fat 41g, Protein 15g, Carbs 4.5g (2 per serving)

Ingredients

1 cup almond flour

½ cup powdered sweetener

1 teaspoon baking powder

1 pinch salt

⅓ cup peanut butter

⅓ cup almond milk

2 large eggs

½ cup chocolate chips

Instructions

Preheat oven to 180C

In a large mixing bowl add all the dry ingredients apart from the chocolate chips mix well

Add the almond milk and peanut butter, stir until combined

Add in 1 egg at a time, incorporating each fully.

Finally, add the chocolate chips and stir to combine

Spray muffin tins with non-stick spray

Divide batter until muffin tins are ¾ full

Bake for about 15 minutes or until a knife comes out clean.

Day 7 - Lunch

BLT (Bacon Lettuce & Tomato) wrap with Avocado – serves 1

Prep time 10 minutes, Cooking time 10 minutes

Nutrition per serving: Calories: 640, Fat 56g, Protein 18g, Carbs 6g

Ingredients

3 large lettuce leaves

3 tablespoons mayonnaise

6 strips bacon cooked to liking

½ large tomato thinly sliced

½ avocado peeled and thinly sliced

Salt and pepper to taste

Instructions

Wash and dry lettuce leaves and flatten slightly

Spread 1 tablespoon of mayonnaise on each leaf

Season with salt and pepper

Add 2 slices of bacon to each leaf

Divide avocado slices and place on each leaf

Wrap tightly

Day 7 - Dinner

Shrimp & Mushroom with cheats noodles – Serves 1

Preparation time,15 minutes, cooking time 20 minutes

Nutrition per serving: Calories : 500, Fat 32g, Protein 44g, Carbs 7.5g

Ingredients

6 oz. large shrimp, peeled

8 oz. mushrooms, sliced

1 tablespoon olive oil

1 tablespoon butter

1 large zucchini

¼ cup marinara sauce

 Salt and pepper to taste

2 tablespoon Parmesan cheese

Instructions

In a medium skillet over medium heat, add the olive oil and fry the mushrooms until most of the oil has been soaked up

Add butter and let the mushrooms cook for another 2 – 3 minutes.

Add the shrimp and cook them for about 4 minutes on each side until they go pink

Using a spiralizer makes cheats noodles from the zucchini

Once the shrimp are cooked, add the zucchini noodles and toss for about 2 minutes.

Add the marinara sauce and season with salt and pepper.

Transfer to a serving plate and top with grated parmesan.

Day 8 - Breakfast

Pizza Omelet with pepperoni and mozzarella – Serves 1

Preparation time 15 minutes, cooking time 15 – 20 minutes

Nutrition per serving: Calories : 600, Fat 53g, Protein 32g, Carbs 5g

Ingredients

3 large eggs

1 tablespoon heavy cream

½ oz. pepperoni slices

½ cup shredded mozzarella

Salt and pepper to taste

1 tablespoon of fresh basil

2 strips of bacon

Instructions

Heat a skillet over medium heat, add bacon and cook until desired crispiness, remove and place on one side

In a medium bowl beat the eggs and then add the heavy cream then pour into the skillet, cook until almost done

Add pepperoni to one side of the cooked egg then sprinkle with mozzarella, salt and pepper and basil

Fold the omelet over and cook for a further 1 to two minutes

Serve warm with bacon slices

Day 8 - Lunch

Chicken and Bacon Salad – Serves 1

Prep time 10 minutes, Cooking time 15 minutes

Nutrition per serving: Calories: 600, Fat 48g, Protein 43g, Carbs 2g

Ingredients

1 large hard-boiled egg

4 oz chicken breast sliced

1 cup spinach washed and dried

2 strips of bacon

¼ avocado peeled and diced

1 tablespoon olive oil

½ teaspoon white vinegar

Salt and pepper to taste

Instructions

Boil eggs for 10 minutes then cool in cold water, peel, and chop

Heat a medium skillet over medium heat, add chicken and cook for 3 minutes

Move chicken to side and add bacon pieces, cook until desired crispiness

In a medium bowl rip spinach leaves and add in the bacon, chicken and chopped egg.

Add Avocado then drizzle with vinegar and olive oil then add salt and pepper to taste.

Toss to coat spinach leaves and avocado

Day 8 - Dinner

Spicy Lime Steak – Serves 1

Preparation time 10 minutes, cooking time 20 minutes

Nutrition per serving: Calories: 560, Fat 34g, Protein 52g, Carbs 8g

Ingredients

7 oz. asparagus

8 oz. thin steak

Salt and pepper for seasoning

Sriracha Lime Sauce:

½ lime

1 tablespoon sriracha sauce

½ teaspoon vinegar

Salt and pepper to taste

1 tablespoon olive oil

Instructions

Place a medium skillet over medium heat, fry asparagus for about 10 minutes, toss occasionally to avoid burning

Season the steak with salt and pepper. Broil until done to your liking turn once.

Remove from broiler, cover the steak and let rest for 5 minutes.

In a small bowl, add lime juice, sriracha sauce, salt and pepper with the vinegar, slowly add olive oil while whisking to combine

Slice steak into thin strips, and serve with asparagus, drizzle sauce over the top.

Day 9 - Breakfast

Breakfast Smoothie – Serves 1

Preparation time – 10 minutes

Nutrition per serving: Calories: 500, Fat 39g, Protein 30g, Carbs 4g

Ingredients

1.5 cups almond milk

1 oz spinach

1/2 avocado

1 tablespoon coconut oil

Sweetener to taste

1 scoop vanilla protein powder

Instructions

Combine all the smoothie ingredients in a blender

Blend on high until everything is smooth and creamy.

Day 9 - Lunch

Tuna Avocado Salad – Serves 1

Prep time 10 minutes,

Nutrition per serving: Calories: 508, Fat 34g, Protein 31g, Carbs 5g

Ingredients

4 oz canned tuna in oil or brine drained

½ stalk celery diced

½ avocado diced

2 tablespoon mayonnaise

1 teaspoon mustard

½ teaspoon fresh lemon juice

Salt and pepper to taste

1 hard-boiled egg, peeled and roughly chopped

Instructions

In a medium bowl add the tuna, celery, and avocado.

Add mayonnaise, mustard, lemon juice, and spices.

Add the egg to the tuna salad.

Mix well until combined.

Day 9 - Dinner

Butter Burger

Preparation time 10 minutes, cooking time 20 minutes

Nutrition per serving: Calories: 640, Fat 59g, Protein 24g, Carbs 1g

Ingredients

4 oz ground beef

1 tablespoon butter

Salt and pepper to season

1 slice cheese

1 teaspoon mayonnaise

1 teaspoon paprika

1 tablespoon olive oil

1 large leaf of lettuce

Instructions

In a small bowl season the ground beef with salt, pepper and paprika and mix very well with your hands.

For in to 2 patties and place the butter in the center of 1 patty

Place the second patty on top of the buttered patty then press to seal the edges, the two patties will now become one

In a small skillet over medium heat, add olive oil and the patty and cook for 4 – 5 minutes on each side

When cooked, serve with lettuce leaf and cheese slice, spread with a small amount of mayonnaise.

Day 10 - Breakfast

Sausage and Egg with Cheese – Serves 1

Preparation time: 15 minutes, cooking time 20 minutes

Nutrition per serving: Calories: 574, Fat 49g, Protein 27g, Carbs 1g

Ingredients

3 oz breakfast sausage

1 large egg

1 tablespoon olive oil

1 cheddar cheese slice

 Chives or spring onion for garnish

Instructions

Heat a skillet over medium heat add olive oil, cook sausage until no longer pink

In the same pan cook egg until the desired doneness

Transfer to serving plate

Garnish with chives or green onion

Day 10 - Lunch

Chicken & Broccoli Casserole with Cheddar topping: Serves 2 or 2 portions

Prep time 20 minutes, Cooking time 30 minutes

Nutrition per serving: Calories: 548, Fat 42g, Protein 44g, Carbs 4g

Ingredients

10 oz chicken breast sliced

2 cups broccoli florets fresh or frozen

2 tablespoon olive oil

1/4 cup sour cream

1/4 cup heavy cream

Salt and pepper to taste

1/2 teaspoon oregano

1/2 cup cheddar cheese grated

1 oz pork rinds crushed

Instructions

Preheat the oven to 230C

In a large bowl add chicken, broccoli, olive oil, and sour cream, mix well

Place mixture in greased baking dish

Pour heavy cream on top to cover

Season with salt pepper and oregano

Cover with grated cheddar cheese and sprinkle with crushed pork rinds

Bake for about 20-25 minutes

Day 10 - Dinner

Fish Fillet with Avocado Sauce - Serves 2

Preparation time 10 minutes, cooking time 20 minutes

Nutrition per serving: Calories: 91, Fat 8g, Protein 2g, Carbs 6g

Ingredients

1 small ripe avocado, coarsely chopped

1/4 cup heavy cream

1 tablespoon lime juice

1 clove garlic, minced

1 dash hot sauce

2 tablespoons lemon juice

1 tablespoon light soy sauce

1 teaspoon lemon rind, grated

1 teaspoon Dijon mustard

2 medium fish fillets

1/2 cup pork rinds, crushed

None-stick cooking spray

Instructions

Pre-heat over to 230C

Add avocado, heavy cream, lime juice, garlic and hot sauce to a blender and blend until a creamy texture, set aside

In a small bowl, add lemon juice and zest, light soy sauce with the mustard

Dip fish fillets into lemon juice mixture and coat with crushed pork rinds

Placed on baking tray which is greased with non-stick spray bake for 7 minutes then turn fillets and bake for a further 7 minutes until the fish starts to flake.

Transfer to serving plate and top with avocado sauce.

Day 11 - Breakfast

Fat Coffee – Serves 1

Preparation time 10 minutes

Nutrition per serving: Calories 273, Fat 30g, Carbs and Protein 0g.

Ingredients

1 Cup Coffee

1 Tablespoon Unsalted Butter

1 Tablespoon Coconut Oil

1 Tablespoon Heavy Cream

Instructions

Brew a cup worth of coffee into a blender

Add 1 tablespoon of butter, coconut oil and finally cream

Blend together very well for 20 seconds

Serve immediately

Chicken and Cheat Noodle Soup – Serves 3 or 3 portions

Prep time 20 minutes, Cooking time 30 minutes

Nutrition per serving: Calories: 370, Fat 26g, Protein 23g, Carbs 8g

Ingredients

8 oz. chicken breast thinly sliced

2 tablespoon olive oil

¼ cup sour cream

½ white onion chopped

1 medium carrot chopped

1 stalk celery chopped

1 tablespoon dried oregano

1-quart chicken stock

1 large zucchini

Instructions

In a large pan, heat olive oil over medium heat and cook onion until tender

Add chicken and cook until starting to brown

Add carrots and celery and season with salt, pepper, and oregano cook until soft

Add the chicken stock and bring the mixture to a boil.

Then lower the heat to a simmer, add chicken and cook 20 minutes.

Spiralize the zucchini into thin noodles, add to the soup during the last 2 or 3 minutes of cooking.

Transfer to serving dish and add sour cream

Nutrition is for 1/3 of the recipe.

Day 11 - Dinner

Cheesy Pork Bake – Serves 2

Preparation time 10 minutes, cooking time 30 minutes

Nutrition per serving: Calories: 474, Fat 36g, Protein 30g, Carbs 6g

250g pork steak

3/4 cup heavy cream

6 oz cream cheese, cubed

1/4 cup soy flour

Salt and pepper

1 teaspoon Paprika

Butter to fry in

1/2 tablespoon garlic salt

1/2 cup Parmesan cheese

Instructions

Slice pork steak into thin strips

Mix flour salt and pepper with the paprika

Coat the steak with the seasoned flour

Heat a skillet over medium heat add butter and cook pork until brown

In a small saucepan, heat milk and add cream cheese, garlic salt and half of the Parmesan cheese, mix well until blended.

Place pork pieces in a small baking dish

Cover with sauce and remaining 1/4 cup Parmesan cheese.

Bake at 180c for 20 minutes, or until going golden.

Day 12 - Breakfast

Keto Porridge: Serves 2

Preparation Time: 5 minutes, Cooking time 15 minutes

Nutrition per serving: Calories 572, Fat 50.2g, Protein 14.8g, Carbs 6g

Ingredients

2 tablespoon hemp seeds

¼ cup walnut or pecan chopped

¼ cup flaked coconut

2 tablespoon chia seeds

3/4 cup unsweetened almond milk

¼ cup coconut milk

¼ cup almond butter (roasted)

1 tablespoon extra-virgin coconut oil

½ teaspoon ground turmeric

1 teaspoon honey

pinch ground black pepper

Instructions

Place a skillet over medium heat

Add the chopped nuts, hemp seeds and flaked coconut and roast for 1 -2 minutes' toss to prevent burning.

Once cooked place in a small bowl and set aside

In a small saucepan heat the almond milk, coconut milk, before it comes to a boil remove from the heat, and add the coconut oil, almond butter, chia seeds, turmeric powder, black pepper and sweetener to taste. Mix until well combined and set aside and let stand for 5-10 minutes. Add half of the dry roasted mix from the bowl.

Divide the porridge into serving bowls and top with the remaining dry roast mix. Finally, drizzle with honey. Porridge can be stored in the refrigerator for 2 – 3 days, add dry mix and honey before serving.

Day 12 Lunch

Asian Beef and Coleslaw – Serves 2 or 2 portions

Prep time 10 minutes, Cooking time 20 minutes

Nutrition per serving: Calories: 370, Fat 27g, Protein 24g, Carbs 4g

Ingredients

1 tablespoon olive oil

2 clove garlic crushed

250 g ground beef

5 oz. coleslaw salad mix

1 tablespoon olive oil

1 tablespoon soy sauce

Salt and pepper to taste

1 teaspoon sesame seeds

1 spring onion chopped

Instructions

In a skillet or wok add a little olive oil and heat on medium – high,

Start by heating the olive oil in a large wok and crushing the garlic clove into it. Cook until fragrant.

Add the ground beef and brown for 5 – 10 minutes, break any lumps with a spoon

Once cooked add the coleslaw mix and stir to combine

Add in olive oil and soy sauce.

Stir and let cook for about 5 minutes until coleslaw mix wilts

Season with salt, pepper, and sesame seeds.

Serve with a sprinkle of spring onion

Nutrition is for 1/2 of the recipe.

Deep Dish Pizza Quiche – Serves 4

Preparation time 10 minutes, cooking time 30 minutes

Nutrition per serving: Calories: 302, Fat 24g, Protein 17g, Carbs 3g

Ingredients

2 cups cheddar cheese grated

2 oz cream cheese, softened

2 large eggs

1/4 cup heavy cream

1/8 cup Parmesan

1/4 teaspoon Italian seasoning

1/4 teaspoon garlic powder

1/3 cup pizza sauce,

1 cup mozzarella, torn into small pieces

Instructions

Preheat oven to 200C

In a medium bowl beat together the cream cheese, eggs, parmesan and spices

Spray a 9−inch or larger glass baking dish with oil then add the 2 cups pizza cheese into the dish Pour egg mixture over the cheese.

Bake for 20 - 30 minutes or until eggs are set.

Spread on pizza sauce, mozzarella cheese and favorite toppings.

Bake until bubbly and browning. Let stand 10 minutes before serving

Make sure to adjust carb counts for your favorite toppings you may use.

Week 2 – Snacks

Vanilla Ice Cream – 6 servings

Prep time 10 min, cook time 3-4 hours or overnight

Nutrition per serving: Calories 238, Fat 22.2 g, Protein, 5.1g, Carbs 2.3g

Ingredients

4 large eggs, separated (pasteurized)

¼ teaspoon cream of tartar or apple cider vinegar

½ cup powdered Erythritol or Swerve or another healthy low-carb sweetener

1 ¼ cups heavy whipping cream - chilled

1 tablespoon vanilla extract

Instructions

Separate the egg whites from the egg yolks.

Whisk the egg whites and add the cream of tartar.

As the egg whites thicken, slowly add the powdered Erythritol (sweetener)

Whisk until soft peaks form

In another bowl whisk cream until soft peaks form

In a small bowl beat the eggs yolks and vanilla extract

Fold the eggs whites into the whipped cream

Gently add the egg mixture and combine

Place mixture into a suitable container, and freeze for 3-4 hours, overnight is better

Baked Parsnip Chips – 4 servings

Prep time 20 minutes, cooking time 10 minutes

Nutrition per serving: Calories 45, Fat 2g, Protein 0g, Carbs 4g

Ingredients

2 medium parsnips, peeled and thinly sliced

Oil for frying (your choice)

Salt

Instructions

Preheat oven to 190C

In a bowl add the parsnip pieces and some olive oil, mix by hand to cover all sides of the parsnip

Place on a lined baking sheet (wax paper) leaving space in between

Bake for 6 – 8 minutes until golden brown

Remove from oven and sprinkle with salt

Chocolate Peanut Butter Balls

Prep time 20 minutes, cooking time 10 minutes

Nutrition per serving: Calories 208, Fat 20g, Protein 4.4g, Carbs 1g

Ingredients

1/2 cup coconut oil

1/4 cup unsweetened grated coconut

1/4 cup Cocoa Powder

4 tablespoon. PB Fit Powder (Peanut butter powder)

6 tablespoon shelled hemp seeds

2 tablespoon heavy Cream

1 teaspoon vanilla extract

28 drops Liquid Stevia

Instructions

In a medium bowl, add all the dry ingredients and mix with a fork until combined

Add coconut oil and using hands, mix until everything is combined and starts turning into a paste

Add the heavy cream, vanilla, and liquid stevia. Mix again until everything is combined, and you have a slightly creamy texture

Measure out the unsweetened grated coconut on to a plate.

Form balls using your hands, and then roll in the grated coconut.

Lay on to a baking tray covered in parchment paper.

Place in the freezer for about 30 minutes.

Best serve chilled

Kale Chips

Prep time 10 minutes, cooking time 10 minutes

Nutrition per serving: Calories 110, Fat 5 g, Protein, 5g, Carbs 8g

Ingredients

Kale leaves

Olive Oil

Seasonings of choice

Instructions

Preheat oven to 190C

Wash and dry kale leaves thoroughly

Tear into medium sized pieces

Add to a bowl small amount of oil, kale leaves and spices

Mix with hands to cover all sides of the leaves

Place on baking sheet, leave space in between so air can pass around

Bake for 8 minutes or until crispy (2 minute intervals)

Protein Shake – serves 1

Prep time 5 minutes

Nutrition per serving: Calories 238, Fat 28g, Protein, 29g, Carbs 2g

Ingredients

1 ½ cups almond milk

1 tablespoon coconut oil

1 tablespoon peanut butter

1 scoop chocolate or vanilla protein powder

4 ice cubes

Instructions

Add all the ingredients to a blender

Blend on high until you have a thick creamy consistency

Salted Almond and Coconut Bark – 12 servings

Prep time 15 minutes

Nutrition per serving Calories 161, Fat 15.3g, Protein, 2.6g, Carbs 1.9g

Ingredients

1/2 cup almonds

1/2 cup unsweetened flaked coconut

100g dark chocolate over 70% cacao recommended

1/2 cup coconut butter

1/4 teaspoon sea salt

1 teaspoon vanilla extract

Instructions

Preheat

Heat a skillet on medium high heat, and add the almonds and coconut flakes, fry for about 10 minutes, toss occasionally to prevent burning

In a double boiler, melt the chocolate, and once melted add the coconut butter and vanilla extract

Spread mixture onto a lined baking sheet (wax paper)

Sprinkle almonds and coconut flakes over the surface of the chocolate, push nuts down so they sink into the chocolate

Sprinkle with a little sea salt and place in the refrigerator

Break into pieces when set

Chocolate Cheesecake with Coconut – 8 servings

Prep time 20 minutes, cooking time 10 minutes

Nutrition per serving Calories 161, Fat 15.3g, Protein, 2.6g, Carbs 1.9g

Ingredients

Base

1/4 cup almond meal

1/3 cup Shredded Coconut unsweetened

1 tablespoon powdered sweetener

2 tablespoon Butter melted

Filling

250 g Cream Cheese softened

200 mL Coconut cream

2 tablespoon Cocoa powder

2 tablespoon powdered sweetener

2 teaspoon Coconut Essence

Instructions

Base

Preheat oven to 160C and grease 8 holes of a standard sized muffin tin.

In a small bowl, add the almond meal, coconut, powdered sweetener and the melted butter, using your hands, mix well until everything is combined

Divide the mixture into 8 and press into the holes of the muffin tin. Bake for 10 minutes until golden brown

Filling

In a bowl place, all the ingredients for the filling, mix on low until everything is combined, once combined mix on medium – high for 3 minutes

Spoon the mixture evenly over the cooled bases, Place in the refrigerator for one hour before serving

Week 2 Shopping List

Almonds – 100g, Almond Flour - 250g, Almond meal – 250g, Almond Milk – 500ml

Apple Cider Vinegar – 1 small bottle, Asparagus – 1 bunch, Avocado - 1,

Bacon – 500g, Baking Powder – 20g,

Broccoli – 250g, Butter – 1stick, Canned Tuna – 1 can, Carrots – 1pc, Celery – 1 small bunch, Cheddar Cheese – 250g,

Chia seed – 200g, Chicken breast - 250g , Chicken stock – 500ml, Chives – 1 bunch, Chocolate Chips – 200g

Cocoa Powder100g, Coconut Oil – 150ml, Coffee, Coleslaw salad mix – 1 small pack, Cream Cheese – 120g,

Cream of tartar – 1 small pack, Dark Chocolate – 100g, Dried Oregano – 1 small jar, Eggs - 14, Fish Fillet - 250,

Flaked Coconut – 100g, Fresh Basil – 1 bunch, Lemon - 1, Garlic - 2, Garlic Powder – 1 small pack

Ground Beef – 500g, Heavy Cream – 2 cups, Hemp seeds – 20g, Honey, Hot sauce 1 small bottle.

Italian seasoning – 1 small jar, Jalapeno – 1 tin, Kale – 1 medium pack, Large Shrimp, Lettuce – 1pc, Light soy sauce – 1 small bottle

Lime – 1pc, Liquid Stevia – 1 small bottle, Low carb wrap - 1, Marinara Sauce – 1 pack, Mayonnaise – 1 small jar,

Mozzarella Cheese – 550g, Mushrooms, Mustard, Nonstick cooking spray – 1 can, Olive Oil – 250ml, Paprika – 1 small pack, Parmesan Cheese – 150g, Parsnips – 2pcs , Peanut Butter – 1 smalldish, Peanut Butter Powder,

green Pepper 1 pcs, Pepperoni150g, Pickled Jalapenos 1 can, Pizza Sauce 1 tan, Plum Tomatoes - 4, Pork rinds – 1 pack,

Pork steak – 250g, Powdered Sweetener 1 small pack, Salami – 200g, Salt, Sausage, Sesame seeds – 100 g

Sliced Ham – 100g, Sour Cream -200ml, Soy Flour - 50, Spinach – 1 medium pack, Sriracha Sauce – 1 small bottle, Thin Steak – 250g

Turmeric – 1 small pack, Unsalted butter – 1 stick, Vanilla Extract – 1 small bottle, Vanilla Protein Powder – 1 small can.

Walnut or Pecan – 100g, White Onion – 200g, White Vinegar100 ml, Zucchini – 3 large

Chapter 8 – Week 3 Days 13 - 19

OK, so now you should be getting a good hang of it and I am sure, if you followed the diet to a 'T', you would have seen results by now. So, let's hope this keeps you motivated, and to try the recipes we have for you on week 3.

Day 13 - Breakfast

Fruity Crème Fraiche – serves 2 or 2 portions

Preparation time 10 minutes,

Nutrition per serving: Calories 448, Fat 44.3g, Protein 5.6g, Carbs 6.7g

Ingredients

1 8.5oz package crème Fraiche (Greek yogurt can be used)

2 tablespoon toasted almond flakes

2 tablespoon toasted coconut flakes

6 tablespoon fruit jelly- flavor of choice

Instructions

Place 3 tablespoon of fruit jelly into serving bowl

Add half of the Crème Fraiche to each serving bowl

Top with coconut flakes and almond flakes

Day 13 - Lunch

Beef Patties with Creamy Mustard Sauce – Serves 3, or 3 portions

Prep time 15 minutes, cook time 20 minutes

Nutrition per serving: Calories 509, Fat 34g, Protein 39g, Carbs 5g

Ingredients

500g ground beef

1/2 tablespoon butter

1 tablespoon olive oil

1 spring onion chopped

2 garlic cloves minced

100g mushrooms thinly sliced

Salt and pepper to taste

Mustard Cream Sauce

½ cup heavy cream

½ cup white wine

2 tablespoons Dijon mustard

1 tomato peeled and chopped

1 tablespoons capers

Instructions

Shape beef into 6 patties.

Heat a large skillet over medium – high heat, add butter and melt until it foams

Add spring onion and garlic, sauté until softened, about 30 seconds

Season beef patties with salt and pepper, and cook to the desired degree of doneness, turn once, set aside and keep warm

In the same skillet, add and sauté the mushrooms until limp, then add to the warm beef patties.

To prepare the Sauce, deglaze the pan with dry white wine. Reduce volume by half. Add Dijon mustard, heavy cream, tomato, and capers. Heat slowly until hot but do not boil.

Pour Mustard Cream Sauce over beef and mushrooms

Day 13 - Dinner

Sticky Sesame Beef – Serves 4

Preparation time 10 minutes, cooking time 30 minutes

Nutrition per serving: Calories: 447, Fat 34g, Protein 33g, Carbs 2g

Ingredients

500g sirloin steak, cut into strips

2 tablespoons of honey

3 tablespoons cooking oil, divided

2 tablespoons soy sauce

1/4 teaspoon pepper

3 spring onions thinly sliced

2 garlic cloves, minced

1 tablespoon sesame seeds

Instructions

In a bowl add soy sauce, pepper, onions, garlic, sesame seeds and honey, mix until combined

Add the steak strips, and cover with the sauce, then let sit for 15 minutes

In a skillet over high heat, place 1 ½ tablespoon of olive oil add the contents of the steak and juice, stir fry until the steak becomes brown, or until your desired likeness

Serve immediately over rice or noodles – adjust nutrition levels accordingly

Day 14 - Breakfast

Beef and Pumpkin Hash: Serves 4 or 4 portions

Preparation time: 20 minutes, cooking time 30 minutes

Nutrition per serving: Calories 762, Fat 31.6g, Protein 21g, Carbs 8g

Ingredients

400g ground beef

200g bacon

3 tablespoon butter

500g pumpkin

3 tablespoon fresh parsley

1 tablespoon paprika

½ teaspoon cayenne pepper

pinch freshly ground black pepper

¼ teaspoon salt

Instructions

Cut the pumpkin in half and remove the seeds, Peel and dice the pumpkin into small cubes

Place the beef into a bowl, and keep at room temperature while you prepare the pumpkin

Over medium heat warm 2 tablespoons of butter then reduce the heat, and then add the pumpkin, season with salt and pepper and cook for 10 minutes, stir occasionally to prevent burning

Slice bacon into small strips and cook in a small skillet until slightly crispy

In a bowl, mix beef with paprika, cayenne pepper and season with salt and pepper

In the same pan that cooked the bacon, add the beef and brown for 5 to 10 minutes, stir occasionally to prevent burning, and the beef is evenly cooked. Add bacon pieces and parsley then remove from heat and stir to combine.

Add sautéed pumpkin and combine well together.

Serve immediately.

Day 14 - Lunch

Cheddar Pancakes – Serves 3

Prep time 15 minutes, cook time 20 minutes

Nutrition per serving: Calories 272, Fat 23g, Protein 14g, Carbs 2g

Ingredients

4 oz Cheddar cheese grated

2 large egg yolks, beaten

1 teaspoons butter

1/2 cup sour cream

1/2 teaspoon salt

1 teaspoons thyme

1/4 teaspoon dry mustard

1 tablespoons unflavored protein powder

Instructions

In a medium bowl add cheddar cheese, sour cream, and egg yolks, mix well

In a small bowl add the protein powder, salt, thyme and dry mustard, mix well

Add to cheese and sour cream mixture

Heat a medium skillet over medium heat, add butter and melt

Add batter by the tablespoon into the skillet, maybe 3 or 4 at once

Cook until lightly brown on the bottom, and then turn to cook until golden

Serve immediately.

Day 14 - Dinner

Southwest Steak Sizzler – Serves 4

Preparation time 10 minutes, cooking time 30 minutes

Nutrition per serving: Calories: 350, Fat 31g, Protein 28g, Carbs 2g

Ingredients

Marinade

2 tablespoons dry white wine

1 teaspoon olive oil

1/8 teaspoon hot pepper sauce

2 tablespoons light soy sauce

1 clove garlic, minced

Cooking Mixture

500g beef steaks

2 cloves garlic minced

1/2 cup white onion chopped

1/4 cup green pepper chopped

1/2 teaspoon cumin

1/4 teaspoon oregano

Instructions

In a medium bowl add the marinade ingredients, add steaks to the bowl, cover with cling wrap and refrigerate for 30 minutes, ideally overnight.

Add 1 tablespoon of olive oil to a skillet over medium heat, sauté the garlic, onion, green pepper, cumin and oregano on moderate heat, stirring occasionally for 10 minutes.

Taste, and add garlic salt if needed.

Add steaks and cook for 5 minutes each side, cook until done or to your desired liking

Serve sizzling with your choice of sides, adjust nutrition info accordingly.

Day 15 - Breakfast

Spiced Pumpkin Waffles – Serves 2 (4 waffles)

Preparation time 10 minutes, cooking time 15 minutes

Nutrition per serving: Calories 337, Fat 26.1g, Protein 18.2g, Carbs 4.5g

Ingredients

2 large eggs

2 tablespoon butter

2 tablespoon heavy cream

½ teaspoon of cinnamon powder

¼ cup pumpkin purée

1 scoop whey protein powder, vanilla or plain

1 ½ tablespoon coconut flour or almond flour

1 teaspoon pumpkin pie spice mix

¼ teaspoon baking soda

2 tablespoon powdered sweetener

3-4 drops vanilla extract

Instructions

In a bowl, add eggs and whisk them with the coconut oil, sweetener, and vanilla extract.

Add pureed pumpkin and cream, and whisk until smooth

Add dry ingredients, and beat until well combined.

Preheat waffle maker and cook mixture according to the waffle iron directions.

Day 15 - Lunch

Chicken and Mushroom Soup – Serves 2

Prep time 15 minutes, cook time 20 minutes

Nutrition per serving: Calories 272, Fat 33g, Protein 41g, Carbs 4g

Ingredients

250g pound chicken breast thinly sliced

2 cups chicken stock

1 cup fresh mushrooms roughly chopped

4 tablespoons sesame oil

2 tablespoons Sherry

2 tablespoons fresh parsley roughly chopped

Salt and pepper to taste

Instructions

Thinly slice the chicken breast

In a medium, pan bring to a boil the chicken stock and add the chicken and mushrooms

When the soup starts to boil again and all of the ingredients float to the top, remove from heat.

Add the sesame oil and sherry and taste for seasoning. Add salt and pepper if necessary.

Serve in individual soup bowls, and sprinkle the parsley on top.

Day 15 - Dinner

Wagon Wheel Sausage Pie – Serves 4

Preparation time 10 minutes, cooking time 30 minutes

Nutrition per serving: Calories: 397, Fat 34g, Protein 14g, Carbs 5g

Ingredients

8 oz sausage

8 oz cream cheese

2 eggs

1/3 cup heavy cream

3 cups shredded zucchini

1/2 cup spring onions, chopped roughly

2 tablespoons heavy cream

Salt and pepper to taste

3/4 cup baking mix

Instructions

Preheat oven to 205C

Preheat a skillet over medium heat, cook sausage in their own oil until cooked all the way through, and not pink.

Mix together baking mix, cream and eggs, and pour mixture around sausages.

Add salt and pepper to taste

Arrange sausages in a spoke pattern in the dish.

Pour mix over the sausages, and cook uncovered for 30 minutes

Day 16 - Breakfast

All day Breakfast – Serves 1

Preparation time 15 minutes, cooking time 15 minutes

Nutrition per serving: Calories 489, Fat 41.3g, Protein 19.5g, Carbs 6.6g

Ingredients

1 large egg

3 medium bacon slices

150g mushrooms

½ avocado

1 tablespoon butter

Salt and pepper to taste

Instructions

Place a skillet over medium heat, add a bit of butter then add the mushrooms top side down

Sprinkle with salt and pepper to season, and cook for about 8 minutes

While the mushrooms are cooking, add butter to another small pan and fry the bacon and egg to your liking.

Transfer to serving plate along with the avocado.

Day 16 - Lunch

Cucumber with Tuna Boats – Serves 1

Prep time 15 minutes,

Nutrition per serving: Calories 272, Fat 33g, Protein 41g, Carbs 4g

Ingredients

1 large cucumber

1 can tuna in oil or brine drained

1 hardboiled egg, diced

1/4 cup Cheddar cheese, shredded

1 stick of celery diced

2 tablespoon of cup mayonnaise

2 tablespoons pickle relish

1 tablespoon chopped onion

1 teaspoon lemon juice

1/2 teaspoon salt

Instructions

Cut cucumber in half and then slice into two

Remove seeds, and run a peeler on the bottom side so it will sit flat

In a medium bowl, add all the remaining ingredients and combine.

Spoon mixture into cucumber pieces

Day 16 - Dinner

Steak and Eggs with Seared Tomatoes - Serves 4

Preparation time 15 minutes, cooking time 15 minutes

Nutrition per serving: Calories: 306, Fat 17g, Protein 32g, Carbs 7g

Ingredients

2 tablespoon of olive oil

500g thin steak

Salt and black pepper

4 medium tomatoes

4 large eggs

1tablespoon chopped fresh oregano

Instructions

Heat 1 tablespoon of the oil in a large skillet over medium-high heat

Season the steak with salt and pepper.

Cook the steak, 4 to 5 minutes each side.

Remove from skillet and let rest for 5 minutes, then slice

Add the tomatoes to the skillet cut-side down, cook until browned, 2 to 3 minutes.

Add oil to the skillet, and cook the eggs covered to your desired doneness, 2 to 4 minutes Sprinkle the tomatoes and eggs with the oregano and salt and pepper.

Serve with the steak.

Day 17 - Breakfast

Whipped Coconut Cream with Fresh Berries – serves 4 or 4 portions

Preparation time 10 minutes

Nutrition per serving: Calories 155, Fat 12g, Protein, 2.1g, Carbs 8.5g

Instructions

4 cups fresh berries of your choice

5 fresh mint leaves, plus more for garnish

1 can full-fat coconut milk, chilled

2 teaspoon vanilla

1 teaspoon honey per serving

Instructions

Wash and divide the berries into serving bowls

Finely chop the fresh mint leaves, and sprinkle on the fruits

Open the can of chilled coconut milk, and use a spoon to scoop out the contents of the can into a medium bowl. Discard any juice or save it for another dish.

Add the vanilla extract

Using a mixer (hand mixer ideal) slowly beat the coconut cream, after about 1 minute add honey for sweetness, continue mixing until the coconut cream becomes fluffy.

Serve immediately with the berries

Garnish with extra mint if required.

Day 17 - Lunch

Sausage Frittata – Serves 2 or 2 servings

Prep time 15 minutes, cook time 30 minutes

Nutrition per serving: Calories 535, Fat 42g, Protein 31g, Carbs 6g

Ingredients

4 oz sausage broken into pieces

1/2 onion, chopped

2 garlic cloves minced

1/4 cup ricotta

1/4 cup heavy cream

2 eggs beaten

1/4 teaspoon cayenne

1/8 cup salsa

½ cup Cheddar cheese grated

Salt to taste

¼ cup sour cream

Instructions

Pre-Heat oven to 180C

In an oven-safe skillet, sauté the onions and garlic for about 30 – 40 seconds. Add broken up sausage, and cook until no longer pink.

In a medium bowl, add heavy cream crumbled ricotta cheese, beaten eggs, salsa and cayenne pepper then pour over sausage pieces

Place skillet into oven and bake for 20 minutes until starting to firm

Remove from oven and top with grated cheese.

Place under broiler until cheese melts and is golden.

Allow to cool slightly before slicing, and serve with sour cream

Day 17 – Dinner

Omelet with Pesto and Feta Cheese – serves 1

Prep time 10 minutes, cook time 10 minutes

Nutrition per serving: Calories 570, Fat 46g, Protein 30g, Carbs 2.5g

Ingredients

3 eggs

1 tablespoon butter

1 tablespoon heavy cream

1 oz. feta cheese

1 tablespoon pesto

Salt and pepper to taste

Instructions

In a medium bowl, whisk the eggs with the heavy cream

In a medium sized Skillet over medium heat, melt the butter and then add the egg mixture

Cook until almost done.

Crumble feta cheese onto one half of the omelet and spread a tablespoon of pesto onto the cheese

Fold the omelet over and cook for another 4 to 5 minutes until the cheese melts

Serve with more feta and fresh herbs

Day 18 - Breakfast

Chai Spice Mug Cake – Serves 1

Preparation time 10 minutes, cooking time

Nutrition per serving: Calories 439, Fat 42g, Protein 12g, Carbs 4 g,

Ingredients

1 Large Egg

2 Tablespoon. Butter

2 Tablespoon Almond Flour

1 Tablespoon Sweetener of choice

7 Drops Liquid Stevia

1/2 teaspoon. Baking Powder

1/4 teaspoon Cinnamon

1/4 teaspoon Ginger

1/4 teaspoon Cloves

1/4 teaspoon Vanilla Extract

Instructions

Mix all room temperature ingredients together in a large mug.

Microwave on high for 70 seconds.

Eat directly from the mug, or place on serving plate

Turn cup upside down and lightly bang it against a plate.

Optional – top with a little heavy cream

Day 18 - Lunch

Zucchini Hash Browns – Serves 2 or 2 portions

Prep time 15 minutes, cook time 30 minutes

Nutrition per serving: Calories 213, Fat 17g, Protein 10g, Carbs 6g

Ingredients

1 1/2 pounds' zucchini

1/2 teaspoon salt

2 eggs

¼ cup Parmesan cheese, grated

2 garlic clove, minced or pressed

1/8 cup butter

Instructions

Coarsely shred zucchini (about 4 cups) into a medium bowl, add salt and let it stand for 15 minutes. Squeeze excess moisture with hands

Add eggs, cheese and garlic

In a large skillet over medium heat, add 2 tablespoons of butter

Mound about 2 tablespoons of mixture and flatten in a skillet to form a patty. Add patties to the pan, but avoid overcrowding

Cook until golden then turn once and cook until golden about 6 – 8 minutes

Repeat until mixture is finished, add more butter to the pan if needed.

Day 18 - Dinner

Ham and Asparagus Bake – Serves 2 or 2 portions

Prep time 15 minutes, cooking time 30 minutes

Nutrition per serving: Calories 208, Fat 15g, Protein 15g, Carbs 2g

Ingredients

200g cooked ham chopped

3 oz cheddar cheese grated

2 tablespoons butter

¼ cup white onion diced

250g Asparagus

3 large eggs

1/3 cup heavy cream

1 teaspoon dried mustard

Salt and pepper to taste

Instructions

Preheat oven to 180C

In a large skillet over medium heat add butter, once melted, add onion, asparagus and ham, cook for about 3 minutes

In a medium bowl mix eggs, cream, and seasonings

In a medium baking dish add Asparagus mixture and then pour over egg mixture and bake for 20 minutes

Sprinkle with grated cheese and bake an additional 10 minutes or until cheese starts to brown.

Day 19 - Breakfast

Creamy Coffee Shake – Serves 1

Preparation time 5 minutes

Nutrition per serving: Calories: 425, Fat 38, Protein 25g, Carbs 1g

Ingredients

1 cup brewed coffee

¼ cup heavy cream

1 tablespoon coconut oil

1 scoop low carb, vanilla protein powder

Instructions

Add the brewed coffee to a blender

Add coconut oil, protein powder, and heavy cream

Blend on high for about 20 seconds or until well mixed

Day 19 - Lunch

Spicy Bacon and Brussels Serves 2 or 2 portions

Preparation time 15 minutes, cooking time 30 minutes

Nutrition per serving: Calories: 278, Fat 21g, Protein 15g, Carbs 4g

Ingredients

250g brussels sprouts

2 tablespoon olive oil

4 strips bacon

Salt and pepper

½ tablespoon cayenne pepper

Instructions

Preheat oven to 190C

Trim the sprouts, if large cut them in half

In a medium bowl toss sprouts with olive oil, salt and pepper, cayenne pepper

Place sprouts on a greased baking sheet and bake for 30 minutes, shake the baking tray after 15 minutes to cook evenly

In a medium skillet over medium heat, cook bacon until desired crispiness, once cooked cut into bite sized pieces

Remove sprouts from the oven and toss in a large bowl with the bacon pieces

Day 19 - Dinner

Sweet & Spicy Chicken with Shrimp – Serves 2

Preparation time 10 minutes, cooking time 20 minutes

Nutrition per serving: Calories: 591, Fat 39g, Protein 50 g, Carbs 3g

Ingredients

2 boneless chicken breasts

20 large shrimp

250g mushrooms

2 handfuls fresh spinach

1/4 cup mayonnaise

2 tablespoon sriracha

1 tablespoon coconut oil

2 teaspoon lime juice

1 teaspoon salt and pepper

1 teaspoon garlic powder

1/2 teaspoon crushed red pepper

1/2 teaspoon paprika

1/2 teaspoon powdered sweetener or honey

1 spring onion

Instructions

Tenderize chicken between plastic wrap until 1 inch thickness, season with salt and pepper and garlic powder

In a skillet over medium heat, add oil and chicken breasts, cook for 8 minutes and then turn, reduce heat and cover

Slice mushrooms and add to the chicken, season with salt and pepper, add oil if needed.

In a small bowl add mayonnaise, sriracha, powdered sweetener or honey, whisk to combine

Heat pan over medium heat, and place shrimp in one layer, add sauce and toss to cover, cook for 3 minutes until shrimp are pink, stir occasionally

When cooked, remove from heat and add the lime juice, and then toss to cover all the shrimp

Place spinach on serving plates with cooked mushrooms, add chicken, shrimp and top with sauce

Sprinkle with spring onion to garnish

Week 3 - Snacks

Raspberry Lemon Popsicles – 6 popsicles

Prep time 15 minutes, chilling time 2 – 3 hours

Nutrition per serving: Calories 151, Fat 16g, Protein 0.5g, Carbs 2g

Ingredients

100g Raspberries or any other in season berries

Lemon juice of half a lemon

1/4 cup coconut oil

1 cup Coconut Milk (carton type)

1/4 cup Sour Cream

1/4 cup Heavy Cream

1/2 teaspoon. Guar Gum

20 drops Liquid Stevia

Instructions

Add all ingredients into a container, and use an immersion blender to blend the mixture together, a normal blender can also be used.

Blend on high until all the berries are mixed with the other ingredients

Strain the mixture to remove any seeds

Pour the mixture into popsicle molds and freeze for a minimum of 2 hours

Run the mold under hot water for a few seconds to loosen the popsicles.

Jalapeno Popper Balls 3 servings

Prep time 15 minutes, cooking time 10

Nutrition per serving: Calories 207, Fat 1.5g, Protein 4.8g, Carbs 1.5g

Ingredients

3 oz Cream cheese

3 slices Bacon

1 medium Jalapeno Pepper

1/2 teaspoon dried Parsley

1/4 teaspoon onion Powder

1/4 teaspoon garlic Powder

Salt and Pepper to taste

Instructions

Place a skillet over medium heat and fry bacon until really crispy

Remove bacon and set aside, but keep the remaining grease for later use.

Slice and de-seed a jalapeno pepper, then dice finely

In a bowl add the cream cheese, jalapeno and spices, season with salt and pepper then mix well

Add the remaining bacon fat, and mix together until a solid ball is formed.

Crumble bacon onto a plate.

Roll cream cheese mixture into 3 balls using your hand, then roll the balls into the crumbled bacon to cover.

Maple Pecan Bars – 12 servings

Prep time 15 minutes, cooking time 10

Nutrition per serving: Calories 303, Fat 30.5g, Protein 4.9g, Carbs 2g

Ingredients

2 cups Pecan Halves

1 cup Almond Flour

1/2 cup Golden Flaxseed Meal

1/2 cup Unsweetened grated coconut

1/2 cup coconut oil

1/4 cup Maple syrup

25 drops Liquid Stevia

Instructions

Pre-heat oven to 190C

Heat a skillet over medium-high heat, add pecan halves and toast for 6-8 minutes or until they start to become aromatic

Remove from skillet and allow to cool, place pecans into Ziploc bag and crush with rolling pin

In a bowl add all the dry ingredients and mix with fork to combine

Add the crushed pecans and mix together again.

Add the coconut oil and maple syrup with the liquid stevia, mix well until a crumbly dough is formed

Press the dough into a 11x7 baking dish

Bake for 20-25 minutes or until the edges are starting to brown

Remove from the oven, when partially cooled add to refrigerator for 1 hour

Cut into 12 slices, and remove using a spatula.

Corndog Muffins – 20 servings

Prep time 15 minutes, cooking time 10

Nutrition per serving: Calories 79, Fat 6.8g, Protein 2.4g, Carbs 0.7g

Ingredients

1/2 cup Almond Flour

1/2 cup Flaxseed Meal

1 tablespoon. Psyllium Husk Powder

3 tablespoon powdered sweetener

1/4 teaspoon salt

1/4 teaspoon Baking Powder

1/4 cup Butter melted

1 large Egg

1/3 cup Sour Cream

1/4 cup Coconut Milk

3 hot dogs

Instructions

Pre-heat oven to 190C.

In a bowl mix all the dry ingredients

Add the egg, sour cream, and butter, then mix well until all combined

When mixed, add the coconut milk and continue mixing until batter forms

Divide the batter between 20 greased muffin holes

Cut the hot dogs into pieces, and place a piece into each muffin hole

Bake for 12 minutes and then place under broiler for 1 – 2 minutes until the tops start to brown

Serve up with dipping sauce of choice

Buckeye Cookies – 12 portions

Prep time 15 minutes, cooking time 10

Nutrition per serving: Calories 148, Fat 13.6g, Protein 2.5g, Carbs 4.4g

Ingredients

2 1/2 Cups Almond Flour

1/2 Cup Peanut Butter

1/4 Cup Coconut Oil

1/4 Cup powdered sweetener

3 Tablespoon Maple Syrup

1 Tablespoon Vanilla Extract

1 1/2 teaspoon Baking Powder

1/2 teaspoon Salt

3 – 4 squares dark chocolate 70% cacao and above

Instructions

Preheat oven to 180C

In a bowl add almond flour, powdered sweetener, baking powder and salt, mix well

In a separate bowl add coconut oil, peanut butter, maple syrup, and vanilla extract, mix well with hand mixer or whisk

Sift the dry ingredients into the wet ingredient bowl, mix well until a crumbled dough.

Using your hands mix together and form into a ball, wrap into plastic and chill for 30 minutes

Cut chocolate pieces into small chunks, 1 to 2 pieces for each cookie.

Remove dough and roll into 20 small balls and press chocolate pieces into the dough.

Press the dough into a tablespoon to give a consistent shape and size

Lay on a lined baking sheet 1 inch apart

Bake for 15 minutes or until going golden brown

Microwave Brownies

Prep time 15 minutes, cooking time 10 minutes

Nutrition per serving: Calories 105, Fat 9g, Protein 7g, Carbs 3g

Ingredients

1 Tablespoon Almond Butter

1 Tablespoon. Beaten Egg White

1 teaspoon unsweetened cocoa Powder

1/8 teaspoon. Vanilla Extract

3 Drops Liquid Stevia

Pinch of baking soda

Pinch of salt

Instructions

In a small bowl add the egg whites and whisk until frothy

Add all the ingredients to a mug, and mix well with a fork

Place in the microwave and cook for 40 seconds (microwaves are not the same, this time can be different)

Remove from microwave and cover with topping of your choice.

Peanut Butter Cookies – 12 portions

Prep time 15 minutes, cooking time 15

Nutrition per serving: Calories 97, Fat 1.5g, Protein 2.4g, Carbs 1.5g

Ingredients

1/2 Cup Natural Peanut Butter

1/3 Cup powdered sweetener

1/3 Cup Coconut Flour

1/4 Cup Flaxseed Meal

5 Tablespoon Salted Butter

1 Large Egg

1 Tablespoon Heavy Whipping Cream

1 teaspoon Baking Powder

1/4 teaspoon Baking Soda

Instructions

Preheat oven to 180C

In a bowl add soft butter and peanut butter, add cream and mix thoroughly.

Add flax seed and coconut flour, mix well until consistency is similar to dough

Add powdered sweetener, baking soda and baking powder, mix well and add egg

Mix well until you have a creamy pliable texture

Roll the mixture into balls, and place on a lined baking tray 1 inch apart, press dough to flatten slightly

Bake for 15 minutes until edges are starting to brown, let cool completely before moving.

Snickerdoodles – 14 servings

Prep time 15 minutes, cooking time 10 minutes

Nutrition per serving: Calories 97, Fat 1.5g, Protein 2.4g, Carbs 1.5g

Ingredients

2 Cups Almond Flour

1/4 Cup Coconut Oil

1/4 Cup Maple Syrup

1 Tablespoon Vanilla extract

1/4 teaspoon Baking Soda

7 Drops Liquid Stevia

Pinch of Salt

Topping

2 tablespoon cinnamon

2 tablespoon powdered sweetener

Instructions

Preheat oven to 180C

In a bowl add coconut oil, maple syrup, vanilla extract and liquid stevia - mix well

In a separate bowl add almond flour, baking soda and a pinch of salt

Add wet ingredients to dry ingredients, and mix until a dough is formed

In a small dish mix cinnamon and powdered sweetener

Roll dough into balls, and then roll into the cinnamon mixture and flatten to give the cracked surface

Place on a baking tray 1 inch apart

Bake for 10 minutes

Remove from oven and cool before serving

Week 3 Shopping List

Almond flakes – 20g, Almond Butter – 1 small jar, Almond flour 750g,

Almond Milk –, 300ml Asparagus – 250g, Avocado – 1, Bacon – 500g,

baking mix – 1 pack, baking soda – 1 small pack, Beef steak – 1500g

Boneless chicken breast – 750, Brussels sprouts – 100g, Butter – 1 stick

Canned tuna – 1 can, Capers 1 small tin, Cayenne pepper – 1 small jar,

Celery – 1 bunch, Cheddar cheese - 250, Cloves 1 small jar, Coconut flakes – 50g, Coconut milk – 250ml

Coconut oil – 300ml, Cooked ham – 100g, Cooking oil – 100ml, Cream cheese - 250g, Crème Fraiche – 250g

Cucumber – 1 pc, Cumin – 75g, Dark chocolate, - 50g, Dijon mustard – 1 small jar

Dried parsley – 1 small jar, Dry mustard – 1 small pack, Eggs - 25, Feta cheese – 250g

Flaxseed meal – 20g, Fresh or frozen berries – 100g, Fresh parsley – 1 bunch

Fresh spinach – 1 bunch, Fruit jelly – 1 small jar, Garlic – 2 , Garlic powder – 1 small jar, Ginger – 1 pc

Grated coconut – 20g, Green pepper, Ground beef – 900g, Guar gum – 1 small pack

Heavy cream – 500ml, Honey – 1 small jar, Hot dogs – 3pcs, Hot pepper sauce – 1 small bottle

Jalapeno - 1, Lemon – 1pc, Lime – 1pc, Liquid stevia – 1 small bottle, Maple syrup – 50ml

Mayonnaise – 1small jar, Mint leaves – 1 bunch, Mushrooms -250g, Mustard – 1 teaspoon

Mustard cream sauce – 1 pack, Olive oil – 1 small bottle, Onion powder – 1 small jar

Oregano – 1 small jar, Paprika – 1 small jar, Parsley – 1 bunch,

Peanut butter – 1 small jar, Pecans – 100g, Pesto 1 small jar

Pickle relish – 1 small jar, Powdered sweetener – 250g, Protein powder – 500g

Psyllium husk powder – 20g, Pumpkin – 500g, Pumpkin puree – 1 small jar

Pumpkin spice mix – 1 pack, Red pepper flakes – 50g, Ricotta cheese – 100g

Salsa – 1 small jar, Salt and Pepper, Sausage – 259g, Sesame seeds – 25g

Sherry – 1 small bottle, Shrimp – 20pcs, Sour cream – 250ml, Soy sauce – 1 small bottle, Spinach – 1 pack, Spring onion – 1 small bunch

Sriracha – 1 bottle, Thyme – 1 small bunch, Tomato – 5pcs, Vanilla extract – 1 bottle, White wine – 250ml, White Vinegar – 1 Small bottle, White Onion – 2pcs

Zucchini – 2kg

Conclusion

If you are reading this, I would like to thank you very much. The content I have provided you with, is a no frills approach of everything you need to know whilst on the Keto diet. It can be a life changing decision to undertake. This is the reason; this information should be made available to everyone who can benefit.

You may have decided to try this diet for yourself, and as you will see, I have based it on 19 days. This should be achievable for most people, I have also structured the meal plans and included snacks, so any temptation to quit will be minimized. The benefits of the Keto diet increases more all the time, it is not a fad diet as many are, it took nearly 100 years to arrive at the point we are now at, so it has surely stood the test of time. Join the 1000's of people who have already tried, and benefited from the Keto Diet.

-- Gloria Day

Made in the USA
Monee, IL
17 November 2022

17980639R00059